MAN, MEDICINE AND MORALITY

By the same author

Published by Faber and Faber
    Patients as People
    How to learn Medicine
    Medical Misfortunes of the Slocombe Family
    (With C. W. Bartley)

Published by Cambridge University Press and republished by Gregg Press Ltd
    Stephen Hales. An Eighteenth-Century Biography

Published by Pitman Medical Publishing Company
    The London. A Study in the Voluntary Hospital System
            Vol. I   1740–1840
            Vol. II. 1840–1948
    Clinical Medicine. The Modern Approach

Published by Penguin Books
    Human Disease. A Pelican Medical book

Edited by the author and published by Hutchinsons
    Old Contemptible A personal narrative. Harry Beaumont

Man, Medicine and Morality

A. E. CLARK-KENNEDY

ARCHON BOOKS
Hamden, Connecticut

This edition first published
in the United States by Archon Books,
Hamden, Connecticut, 1969

SBN 208 00972 8

Printed in Great Britain

CONTENTS

Acknowledgements   *page* 9

Prologue   11

I. The Body   15

II. The Genesis of the Body   23

III. Hormones and the Nervous System   34

IV. Body-Mind   59

V. Attitude to Life   76

VI. Functional Disorders   92

VII. Organic Disease   108

VIII. Health, Society, Law   131

IX. Patient, Doctor, State   153

X. Problems Relating to Death   190

Index   207

7

ACKNOWLEDGEMENTS

Often, both before and after I started to write this book, I discussed many of the subjects and problems on which I have touched with colleagues, too numerous to mention by name, both at the London Hospital and at Corpus Christi College, Cambridge, but at the latter I would express my particular indebtedness to Dr. Michael Tanner (philosophy), Dr. Richard Bainbridge (zoology) who read part of, and Chancellor the Rev. Evelyn Garth Moore (law) who read the whole of, my manuscript and discussed many points with me in detail. I am also grateful to Professor Leslie Banks, Professor of Human Ecology in the University, and to Dr. Roy Goulding of the Poisons Reference Department, Guy's Hospital; also to Dr. P. Macdonald Tow (neuro-psychology), at one time my student, whose criticism has been invaluable, and to Dr. Christopher Bartley, Physician to the Lambeth Hospital, for many years my medical registrar at 'the London'. But all opinions expressed, and any errors in the statement of fact or theory, must rest squarely at my door. I also wish to acknowledge yet again the unfailing co-operation of my secretary, Mrs. Dorothy Chapple.

A. E. CLARK-KENNEDY

Cambridge
11th November 1968

PROLOGUE

On an historic occasion in the House of Commons in the eighteenth century a certain Mr. Dunning rose to move that 'the power of the Crown has increased, is increasing and ought to be reduced'. Today, in the later twentieth century, it is tempting to parody these words in relation to an important component of the social scene. The power of medicine over human lives and minds 'has increased and is increasing', and, it can be confidently added, is bound to increase, with mounting speed, still further. Whether this fast-growing power 'ought to be reduced' (there is always danger in power), whether doctors are going too far in playing tricks with nature and 'monkeying' with the human body, whether we are losing all sense of personal integrity and human decency in our instinctive desire to live on, whether we are becoming slaves of science rather than masters of our own inventions, is a matter of opinion. But, as to the increasing power of doctors over human lives and minds, there can be no doubt whatever.

Maternal and infant mortality have been reduced by antenatal and post-natal care. Deficiency disease is prevented, and children protected against the serious infections. Bacterial diseases are treated with antibiotics, and even cancer can often be cured by a combination of surgery, X-rays and endocrine therapy. The expectation of life at all ages has been raised. Far more people now live out their allotted span. Average age has increased, and in many countries population will outstrip food supply, unless modern methods of birth control are adopted, or new methods of food production are implemented and others invented.

Further, during the last decade, the practice of medicine has taken an unexpected turn, and now it sometimes seems difficult to see where medicine ends and science fiction begins. Pregnancy can be prevented by taking a pill. A woman can be artificially inseminated, and it would be possible to breed the entire human race from a small number of selected males. The mind can be influenced in new ways with drugs. Personality can be altered by operation on the brain. Not only have the blood groups been discovered, and transfusion rendered safe, but corneal tissue can be grafted, conserving sight, and for some time it has been possible to transplant a kidney from one man into another. Now the heart has been taken out of a dead man, and used to replace that of a living man in whom it has been made to beat, keeping him alive. Further, even if breathing and circulation stop, a man is not necessarily dead. He can sometimes be rescued from the grave by modern methods of resuscitation.

Most of this is common knowledge, and transplant surgery, exciting the imagination of the public, has gained wide publicity. Indeed, medicine has long ceased to be something strange and mysterious which the layman could not understand, and about which he was not expected to ask questions. Rather, he now demands to know what the doctor does, and when and why and how he does it. So the functions of the body, the working of the mind, the most recent discoveries, the latest remedies, the gravest problems, are freely discussed in the popular press, broadcast on the air, and dramatized on the television screen.

Mr. Dunning went on to move that the power of the Crown should be reduced but no one would suggest that modern medicine should be jettisoned. Its success in terms of prolongation of life is far too great for that. On the other hand, the unrestricted use of its increasing power is raising moral problems on which there is no agreement now, and on which agreement is most unlikely ever to be reached in the future. It is also necessitating legislation to protect the public from the risks of its discoveries and abuse of the power which it is putting into human hands. It is also raising financial problems. For the proportion of the national income which can be devoted to health, in view of other claims on it, is of necessity limited, and the cost of modern medicine is steadily rising. A vital question is how this proportion can best be spent.

Further, although better education and modern methods of

communication have resulted in people carrying far more information in their heads than they did, the total corpus of acquired knowledge has grown so great of recent years that a man can now only compass a much smaller fraction of it, and in medicine this has compelled increasing specialization. While the general practitioner knows more and more about less and less, the specialist is coming to know less and less about progressively more and more.

What therefore seemed to me wanted was a straightforward account of the natural phenomenon of disease (with which everyone collides to some extent), the problems of practice and the moral, legal and financial questions precipitated by it, set out in relation to the conflicting claims of human experience, as reflected in religion, on the one hand, and the modern scientific interpretation of the nature of man, on the other. For medicine raises issues which far transcend the boundaries of science. Some concern values of which it can take no account. Others question the nature of man, and collide with hitherto generally accepted moral standards. 'Weary of myself and sick of asking, what I am and what I ought to be', wrote Matthew Arnold, and although few in this generation are as introspective, both his questions remain pertinent to life in general and relevant to medicine in particular. For *What I am* is a question which science can attempt to answer, and can also claim to have advanced some distance towards it while getting the man sick in body or mind back to, or making him *what he ought to be* is the aim, it can be said, and the object and the end of medical practice.

This book is intended for anyone who touches medicine at any point; for doctors forced apart by specialization and temperament; for nurses and social workers in their respective spheres; for health visitors and psychotherapists; for medical administrators and members of hospital boards; for educationalists, priests, and ministers of religion. But it is also written for any layman prepared to face up to an increasingly difficult social problem, and I have endeavoured to write in such a way as to be intelligible to him. The risk is that, in so doing, when I touch on any subject, and I touch on many, the reader with knowledge of it will think my treatment inadequate, while the layman may still find me hard to follow. But I trust that I have never been superficial, and that I shall at least have always created the right impression. It is not intended to advocate particular points of view. Rather, it attempts to state the views that can be held on the issues raised, asking the right questions without attempting to give authoritative answers to them.

It has not been an easy book to write, and I must have often revealed my ignorance. My defence is that every aspect of human experience must be related in some way to every other, and that unless someone has the courage to do something like this sometimes, we shall lose our way in the mass of knowledge which we are creating. Only a physician perhaps, accustomed to deal with all sorts of situations, and compelled to trespass from time to time in fields in which he has no particular know-ledge, would in fact have had the temerity to attempt anything so difficult; and I am old enough to have watched these prob-lems developing. When I started, a physician was a philosopher or a fool, it was said, by the age of forty. Today medicine has grown so complex that he runs the risk, not of becoming a fool—it is too difficult for that—but of becoming a technician, at a time when it is more than ever important that he should become a philosopher with courage, if the increasing power of medicine is to be used with the necessary restraint.

When I started, the doctor's problem was simple. *Could* he keep Mr. X or Mrs. Y alive? Today it is sometimes much more difficult. *Should* he strive to keep Mr. X or Mrs. Y alive? As the power of modern medicine increases, this problem is bound to recur with increasing force and frequency. Only if doctors exer-cise restraint at times, and the general public learns to acquiesce in it, will the increasing power of medicine continue to be used in the best interests of society.

CHAPTER I

THE BODY

*The human machine—The criteria of life—The chemical
basis of life*

The ordinary man who, divesting himself of all previous ideas,
turns in upon himself, and begins to ask his nature, probably
comes to the conclusion that he is some sort of conjunction of
body and something else which, for lack of any more exact
word, he calls his mind. The former he knows to be made of
more or less solid stuff, and to occupy space in three dimensions.
That which he calls his mind lives in time alone, and is more
elusive, but under it, if he stops to think, he probably includes
consciousness, both of himself and of his environment, which
lapses when he goes to sleep; the capacity to suffer pain and
enjoy pleasure, and to be disturbed by emotion; and his innate
ability to remember past events, learn by practice and experience, think, form judgments and concepts, and scheme and
plan ahead. Further, his mind, as he calls it, can order his body
about, and although the state of his body, as he knows from
experience, can have a profound effect on that which he calls
his mind, he gives pride of place to his mind rather than his
body. *Cogito, ergo sum*, I think, therefore I am, wrote René
Descartes three hundred years ago.

The human machine

The scientist, on the other hand, in endeavouring to answer
this question, tends to start prejudiced in favour of his body. Of
the two it is more amenable to study by induction from observation, and deduction from planned experiment, and from his
point of view it clearly falls into the category of a machine, that
is to say, a device for converting one form of energy into the
one best suited to do the work in hand.

15

All living things are machines in this sense. A green plant is so organized that it converts the energy of sunlight into energy containing substance which enables it to hold water, the object of the exercise being to grow, and thereby compete with its neighbours for the sunlight on which its life depends. An animal is so organized—hence the use of the word *organism* to describe animals in general—that it gets the energy it needs from the sun (all energy other than intra-atomic comes from the sun) second-hand by eating plants or other animals, and it is also so constituted that it can grow up, live in time, and move about in space. Further, the animal machine is clearly comparable to the internal combustion engine. It explodes a glucose-oxygen mixture in muscles in much the same way that a motor car, which gets a man about more quickly than his legs, explodes a petrol-oxygen mixture in cylinders.

The animal machine is, however, most peculiar compared with any one of man's invention. While a motor car works at high temperature, and has to be kept cool, the animal body works at low temperature, and even during muscular exercise seldom finds that any great problem. This, of course, had need to be since the stuff out of which it is made is easily destroyed by heat. Its ignition system is also different. In a motor car the petrol-oxygen mixture is fired in cylinders at high temperature by an electric spark. In animals the glucose-oxygen mixture is fired at low temperature in muscles by a nervous impulse.

Man walks on two legs, and animals on four. Cars run on wheels. Further, the conversion of the energy liberated in cylinders and muscles, into movement of wheels and legs respectively, is effected by different methods. In the motor car it depends on the sudden liberation of gas which, by its expansion, drives a piston down a cylinder, the movement of which is converted by crank shafts into the rotation of its wheels. In the body it depends on the fact that the chemical energy liberated in muscle leads to immediate swelling, with consequent shortening of that muscle, as a result of which its points of attachment to two bones, loosely connected at a joint, are pulled together. The man-made engine works by compression and expansion. The human machine works by swelling and contraction.

The body is also constructed on quite different principles to

16

those of a man-made machine. The basic stuff out of which it is made is packed into a vast number of more or less similar cells, each one consisting of a central nucleus surrounded by cytoplasm contained within a limiting membrane. The body is in fact made of cells in much the same way that a house is built of bricks. But this analogy must not be stretched too far. Bricks are manufactured separately, and mortared together artificially. They bear no other relationship to each other. The body has arisen by cell division from a single fertilized ovum in the course of which its cells have become specialized, and to some extent altered in appearance, to serve particular functions in relation to its needs as a whole. The gastro-intestinal tract digests our food. The liver prepares it for use. The lungs take in oxygen. The heart circulates the blood, and this carries the end-products of digestion to the liver; urea, the waste product of protein metabolism, to the kidneys; fuel from the liver, and oxygen from the lungs, to the muscles; carbon dioxide, the main waste product of muscular activity, back to the lungs. Further, it is erroneous to think of a multi-cellular organism as built up of independently designed cells like the parts of a machine. Rather, the body is to be compared to a successful business which has been forced into developing special departments by the pressure of its own success. Every cell is related to every other cell, the body as a whole far greater than the sum of its component parts.

The human machine is also self-maintaining in the sense that, provided it is kept supplied with sufficient water, certain inorganic substances, notably iron, calcium and iodine, and food of the right kind, a man does not need to think what he ought to eat in order to maintain himself in health. Appetite, taste, hunger, thirst and sense of repletion ensure that.

The body is to a large extent self-regulating. Tissue protein broken down in daily wear and tear is automatically replaced out of daily protein intake. The end products of muscular activity are excreted as soon as their concentration in the body passes a certain threshold. Like all warm-blooded animals, a man keeps himself at constant temperature, in spite of considerable fluctuations in his external environment, without thinking about it much. If he is tending to get too hot, heat loss is increased by sweating, which leads to rapid evaporation from his skin, a physical phenomenon associated with absorption of heat, and therefore with fall of temperature. (We sweat to keep cool, *not* because we *are* hot.) If he is tending to get too cold, heat production is increased by that rapid type of muscular action which we call shivering. (We shiver to keep warm; *not* because we *are* cold.) Another example of automatic regulation is acidity-alkalinity control. For the body must be kept just alkaline. During muscular exertion the rate of production of carbon dioxide is increased, and the rate and depth of breathing are automatically raised to get rid of it. A man does not need to think how fast and how deep he ought to breathe when running a race. That is determined for him.

The human body is also self-adjusting in the sense that it is potentially capable of adapting itself to many abnormal situations. If one of the valves of the heart begins to leak, the muscle fibres of the chamber behind grow longer and get stronger and maintain the circulation. If the resistance to the flow of blood increases, the muscle of the left ventricle reacts similarly and maintains the circulation. If any hollow tube becomes slowly obstructed, the muscle behind increases in strength and maintains the traffic through it. If a fractured bone re-unites at the wrong angle, its internal structure is automatically re-adapted to the new lines of force prevailing in it. A man, too, quickly readjusts the physiology of his body to working at night, and in modern warfare men adapt themselves to a more or less underground existence.

The body also reacts to potentially dangerous encounters in such a way as to protect itself against injury, and maintain its integrity. The point of a pin, or sudden contact with a hot object, leads to immediate withdrawal of the part affected—reflex action, as this is called. And there are many other protective reflexes of this kind; coughing, to clear the respiratory tract; screwing up the eyes, in anticipation of a blow; vomiting, to protect the gut. These are part of ordinary experience, and depend, as will be seen later, on inborn paths of low resistance in the nervous system.

Further, the body, when self-protection fails, is to a large extent self-repairing. This again is common knowledge. Blood soon clots, and often stops bleeding. If much blood is lost, the marrow steps up production. A clean cut heals by the formation of fibrous tissue. So, too, with bones and nerves. A surgeon does not *mend* a broken bone. He keeps it still and in the right position, with the aid of splints or plaster, while it mends itself by bone formation. A cut nerve also repairs itself in the sense that the central end grows down the old path until anatomical and functional integrity have been restored.

Not only, too, is the human body, like that of all animal bodies, self-maintaining, self-regulating, self-adapting, self-protecting, and to a large extent self-repairing, but again like all others, if it mates, it is also self-reproducing by the same mechanism as that by which it was itself produced, namely, progressive cell division from a fertilized ovum. Indeed, a remarkable thing about life is that the different forms of it, in spite of their diversity, maintain their fixed forms of structure and function so accurately down the generations. Life and living things in general would in fact appear to contravene the second law of thermodynamics or principle of entropy which asserts that, in any system, order tends to give way to disorder, unless controlled by something from without.

All animals exhibit behaviour, and this can be divided into reflex, spontaneous and volitional. Reflex behaviour is predictable. It can be relied upon to occur again and again, as it does in a man-made machine, in response to the same stimulus applied to the same part of the body, depending, as it does, on the passage of an impulse along the same path in the nervous system. Spontaneous behaviour appears to be due to something going on in the man or in the animal unrelated to anything outside it. Except in sleep, or for a definite purpose, neither keeps still for long. A dog is always sniffing about, a man looking round, either Micawber-like hoping something will turn up, or to be certain that there's nothing in the offing. Besides, in both there is the continual consciousness of mere existence, the sense of the passage of time, and in men particularly, memory and the free association of ideas. Volitional behaviour depends on the last of the pecularities of the animal machine, namely, on the existence of consciousness and mind.

For the human machine, and the machinery of the higher animals, permits the development through the brain of consciousness of self and environment. It is on consciousness that experience writes in order to lead, at least in part—everyone must admit that—to the development of an individual mind which, in the case of man, to a large extent governs his behaviour.

The criteria of life

These peculiarities are the accepted criteria of life. If an object occupying space in three dimensions exhibits them, it is deemed to be alive. Nevertheless, it is now possible to construct machines which, up to a point at least, exhibit characteristics hitherto regarded as monopolies of living things, and hitherto attributed to a vital force believed at one time to exist independently of matter, and said to govern their behaviour.

Machines can certainly be made self-regulating. A thermostat is that, and the governor of a steam engine controls its speed. It is also possible to conceive of a machine which, if provided with the necessary materials, could mend itself. A guided missile homes on its target. It would be possible to construct a machine armed with radar which moved about the room avoiding the light, if it were provided with a mechanical eye in the form of a photo-electric cell. The proverbial man from Mars, seeing it walk in and walk out, might well maintain that it must be alive. Further, a computer now does much of the mental work heretofore done by human brains. Indeed, when all the differences between men and machines are boiled down, the basic difference between them turns on their cellular structure, growth by cell division, and more than anything else on the stuff out of which they are made. This latter permits, it seems, all the peculiar manifestations of life, including consciousness and mind. Until man can make this stuff, he will not have created life as we know it, and, until this is made, a fundamental difference remains between men and man-made machines.

The chemical basis of life

The nuclei of all cells consist maintly of nucleo-protein, and now it has been discovered that the most important component of it is desoxyribonucleic acid, called D.N.A. for short. This, it is now also known, is made up of a chain of chemical units called nucleotides. Each of these consists of one of four nitrogen-containing bases, adenine, guanine, thymine and cytosine, combined with a sugar, desoxyribose. In D.N.A., these units are linked together by phosphate like this:

Base 1 — Sugar
    >Phosphate
Base 2 — Sugar
    >Phosphate
Base 3 — Sugar
    >Phosphate
Base 4 — Sugar

Innumerable varieties of D.N.A. therefore exist, on account of the vast number of permutations and combinations of ways in which its constituent bases can be arranged.

D.N.A., it is now known, 'directs' activity in all parts of the cell by sending out chemical 'messengers' which 'tell' them what to do and when to do it. Further, it is also known that these D.N.A. chains are arranged in identical pairs, coiled round each other in double spirals, the so-called double helix, and that these often uncoil and separate, each one then attracting to itself, provided energy is available, the necessary substances from its environment to reconstruct another opposite number for itself, leading to cell division. The one-time concept of an independent vital force responsible for the growth and behaviour of living things has in fact given way to the concept of them all depending on the peculiar way in which certain large molecules, based on carbon and containing nitrogen and phosphorus, behave, but behave, and this is the important point, in strict conformity to the laws which govern matter of all kinds. In short, the old concept of vitalism has shifted its ground, and become respectably chemical. Just as we know that electricity is not a principle of nature, but the way in which matter behaves according to physical laws under certain circumstances, so life, we now know, is not a separate principle either, but the way in which certain molecules behave according to the laws which govern all other molecules as well.

This discovery is likely to have great practical consequences. As our knowledge of the chemistry of the body increases, further advances in both the treatment and prevention of diseases seem bound to follow. There is now no *theoretical* reason why men should not succeed in starting new life in the laboratory, and make new living machines to do his chemical work for him, just as he already uses existing living machines to do much of it, as when he brews beer, bakes bread, or ploughs in a vetch to nitrify the soil. But, although science is fast beginning to describe life in scientific language, it does not provide us with any satisfying explanation of it in terms of our own conceptual experience. In consequence we are left compelled to continue to use human language—for example, directing operations and sending out messengers—to *explain* for our own benefit biological phenomena which science *describes* in terms of the fundamental nature of the universe.

*　　*　　*

The body is a machine made of protein arranged in cells which converts the food it eats into its substance, and oxidizes the rest to provide the necessary energy to keep it warm and enable it to move about. It maintains itself, repairs itself, reacts to change and, if it mates, reproduces itself. Further, it becomes conscious of its environment and of its own existence as a unit of life in time and in space in three dimensions.

CHAPTER II

THE GENESIS OF THE BODY

Germ cells and genes—The genetic plan—D.N.A. and R.N.A.— Development—Variation—The origin of man.

The mind has been intensively studied of recent years both by observation and experiment. But, before trying to give the answer, which modern science would seem to give, to the ordinary man's question *What is my mind*, we must first give some account of the origin of the body and the working of certain aspects of it.

Germ cells and genes

Every living body, and that of everyone who has ever lived, was determined, we now know, by progressive cell division from a single fertilized ovum, the result of fusion of male and female germ cells. The latter, in their turn, were derived from male and female bodies which had already attained maturity.

Spermatozoa and ova, like all cells, both consist of a nucleus and surrounding cytoplasm, the latter containing rod-like structures known as chromosomes. These are arranged in pairs which are said to be homologous, because their members look alike, although pairs differ in their appearance and can be recognized at sight. All the somatic cells of the same species carry the same number of chromosomes. Every species has a characteristic chromosome number. That of man is forty-six. Further, these chromosomes are now known, as the result of breeding experiments, to carry the genes, anatomical units which control the inheritance of many of the characteristics by which animals and plants of the same species, i.e. those capable of interbreeding, differ from one another.

In all ordinary cell divisions, i.e. in those associated with growth and repair, the chromosomes divide with the cell so that their number remains unchanged. At the same time the genes are duplicated, so that each daughter cell is an exact replica in these respects of its parent cell and, reasoning backwards, also of the fertilized ovum whence it was derived. In other words, if a fertilized ovum can be said to contain the plan for the development of the whole body, then every cell in it can be said, as the result of this process, to have been provided with a copy of it, although that cell itself has only carried out its own small part in the scheme for the construction of the body as a whole.

In the two cell divisions leading to the formation of the germ cells, events take a different course to that followed in the formation of somatic cells. This is destined to have profound consequences in respect of individual development.

In the first of these the chromosomes get together in their homologous pairs. Then each one of a pair twists round and embraces the other, allowing lengths of each, containing genes, to cross over from one to the other, a process which occurs at random in the sense that its details cannot be predicted. So, although these chromosome pairs still look the same, they are now different in respect of their gene content. Then, newly constituted in this way, they replicate themselves by dividing longitudinally so that each daughter cell resulting from this division is now identical with the other in respect of their new gene content.

In the second the chromosomes do not replicate themselves. Instead, the homologous pairs break up, one chromosome of each pair now passing, at random in relation to all the other pairs, into one daughter cell, and the other chromosome into the other. The germ cells (gametes) thus formed therefore contain only half the normal number of chromosomes, human germ cells only twenty-three. So, as for n pairs of chromosomes there are 2^n possible combinations of them in respect of each new cell, there are 2 to the power of 23 of them in human germ cells.

When an ovum is fertilized by fusion with a spermatozoon the normal number of chromosomes is restored, and twenty-three new homologous pairs are formed. One chromosome in each new pair is now maternal and the other paternal in origin, each containing genes derived from a man's mother's family and his father's family respectively. So two elements of chance

24

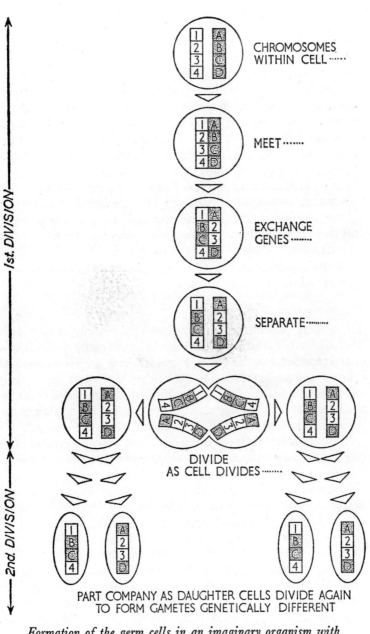

Formation of the germ cells in an imaginary organism with
one pair of homologous chromosomes each carrying four genes,
i.e. A to D *and* 1 to 4

enter into the genesis of a man. In the first place, chance crossing over of genes, followed by the random segregation of the chromosomes in the formation of his parent's germ cells, resulted in all of them differing in gene content among themselves. In the second, chance determined which of his father's spermatozoa, formed in this way, happened to fuse with which of his mother's ova, formed in this way, at his conception. Further, as will be seen in a moment, chance meeting of the two sex chromosomes to form a new homologous pair determined his sex at this moment. Hence the similarity and the wide differences, leaving the possibility of mutation out of account for the moment (p. 30), between children and their parents, and between children of the same parents, identical twins derived from the same fertilized ovum excepted. Hence, too, both the similarities and the wide differences between individuals within the human race.

The genetic plan

These facts provide an anatomical explanation of Mendel's laws of heredity relating to the inheritance of easily recognizable characteristics. For the genes, some of which are dominant and others recessive in relation to each other in their effect on their transmission, are shuffled and reshuffled, like packs of cards, in the formation of the gametes and again in the restoration of the normal chromosome number when an ovum is fertilized.

Many characteristics in domestic animals when crossed with one another are transmitted in accordance with Mendel's laws. Mendelism also applies to man. Colour of hair and eyes, colour vision, and the ability to taste certain substances, are inherited according to Mendel's laws. The transmission of the blood groups is Mendelian, and a number of familial diseases are inherited in this way. Some are due to a dominant gene. Several members of the same family are affected, and cases turn up in every generation. Others rarely affect more than one member, and only appear occasionally. These are due to a recessive gene transmitted down the generations behind the scenes. A few are sex-linked. For sex is determined by two special chromosomes. One of these is large, and known as the X; the other small, and known as the Y. A man's cells contain X *and* Y chromosomes;

a woman's two Y's. When the germ cells are formed, the sex chromosomes part, all gametes containing only an X or only a Y chromosome. Then, if one of the former meets a Y, that conception gives rise to a male. If it meets another Y, it leads to a female.

But there is still a vast unbridged gap in our knowledge between what we now know about the inheritance of odd characteristics, blood groups, familial diseases and determination of sex, on the one hand, and what we know about the inheritance of all the ordinary characteristics of a species, on the other. Although we are able to account for a man's sex, blood group, eye colour, and for colour blindness and many familial diseases, we do not yet know how he manages to inherit his human head and face, his two arms and legs, his hands and feet, his trunk, let alone his heart and guts or, of course, his brain on which his mind develops. Nevertheless, it seems reasonable to suppose that the inheritance of all physical characteristics must be due to complex interaction between large numbers of genes.

We are in fact driven to conclude that, when an ovum is fertilized, a configuration of genes is set up which, environment permitting, proceeds to condition the development of a new unit of human life in all its characteristic aspects. Not only does the meeting of certain chromosomes determine the sex of the individual, and the relationship of certain genes predetermine certain physical features which normally vary among men, but the configuration of genes established at that moment conditions development in such a way that he or she, whichever 'it' is destined to be, develops all the ordinary characteristics of the human species, and also develops them in such a way as to resemble his or her parents, or even his or her remote ancestors, in certain respects. Just, in fact, as St. Paul's Cathedral can be regarded as the product of both the plan engendered in the mind of Christopher Wren and stone dug out of the ground, so the body of every human being that has ever existed, exists today, or will ever exist, must be regarded as having been, being, or destined to be, the product of both a genetic plan laid at its conception and materials derived directly or indirectly from its environment.

There is a fundamental difference however between the plan

for the cathedral, to continue the analogy, as it was drawn out, and the pattern of genes in a fertilized ovum destined, all being well, to result in a new member of the species. Wren had to employ contractors to assemble the necessary materials and builders to put his plan into execution. He also had to tell the builders how to put the cathedral up, when to start building each part in relation to every other part in such a way, for instance, that the sides of the arches met at the right place at the right moment, and the cathedral did not tumble down in the course of its own construction. In short, builders and contractors had to work to his schedule and to his time-table. But the genetic plan for the body contains its own building instructions and its own complicated time-table; and proceeds to execute itself. The plan for the execution of the genetic plan is in fact vested in it, and it is in this extended sense that *genetic plan* must be understood when we refer to it throughout this book.

D.N.A. and R.N.A.

How does the fertilized ovum do it? How does it 'know'—it is difficult to avoid the word—how to convert the glucose and amino acids in its immediate vicinity into its own right protein substance? How does it 'know' when it should divide into two, then into four, and then into eight? How does it 'known' how to produce the right enzyme to do the right thing, at the right speed, at the right place, at the right time, so that differentiation of structure results, and the foundations of the different parts of a human body are laid, and slowly come into being in orderly sequence? How does the detailed time-table for all this come to be vested in the fertilized ovum whence a man is derived? Must we revert to the concept of a vital force, or postulate some form of directional control from without? Or, can it be explained, or at least described, in terms of the general statement already made, to the effect that all manifestations of life are due to the way in which certain molecules behave in obedience to the laws which govern matter?

The answer to that is that it can, and the key substance here would now appear to be another complex long-chained molecule, namely, ribo-nucleic acid, or R.N.A. It is closely allied to D.N.A., the only difference between them being the sugar in the molecule; ribose instead of desoxyribose. (Hence the abbreviations D.N.A. and R.N.A.) They behave differently however. D.N.A. molecules duplicate themselves at each cell division, but stay put in the nucleus, ensuring that a copy of the plan is always handed on. The R.N.A. molecules, formed from D.N.A. in much the same kind of way as that in which R.N.A. duplicates itself, diffuse out into the cytoplasm of the cell. They carry the necessary instructions to start the formation of the enzymes responsible for the chain of chemical reactions which lead to differentiation of structure in accordance with the plan laid at conception. This process must be exceedingly complicated, and we can only claim to possess an inkling as to how it works. It is possible, for instance, to envisage how the right proteins are made. But it is hard to see at present how they get formed in the right order in respect of time, and laid down right in respect of the three dimensions of space. Further, this concept is again descriptive rather than explanatory. But our knowledge is now sufficiently advanced to rule out any need for the concept of a vital force to explain development. The execution of the plan laid at conception, it now seems certain, depends on the peculiar properties of nucleo-protein.

Development

The fertilized ovum divides almost at once. Then each daughter cell divides into two more, making four; then each of these again, making eight, and so on until a mass of several thousand has been formed. Organization of structure now begins as the result of a succession of chemical reactions. Invaginations at places destined to become the head and tail end respectively, meeting in the middle, form the intestinal tract, and differentiate this primitive mass into two layers, ectoderm and endoderm. Each of these now splits to form the two layers of the mesoderm, with the primitive body cavity, represented in the adult by the thoracic and abdominal cavities, between them. The mesoderm gives rise to the bones and muscles, to the heart and vessels, to the kidneys and suprarenals; also to the reproductive glands, the testes or ovaries according to sex. An outgrowth at the front end of the primitive gut gives rise to the lungs; another to the anterior lobe of the pituitary; a third to

MAN, MEDICINE AND MORALITY

the thyroid. The nervous system is formed by an infolding of the ectoderm, the complexities of which at the head end give rise to the brain, while from all parts of it fibres grow out to supply the muscles developed from the mesoderm. Within six weeks the foundation of all the main organs of the body has been laid.

Growth is now mainly a matter of increase in size, and within nine months approximately fifty generations of cell division have resulted by geometrical progression in approximately 2^{50} cells, weighing a total of seven to eight pounds, arranged in the form of a human body. Some organs are already in action. The heart is circulating the blood elaborated by the marrow, and paths for the execution of reflex movement have already been laid down in the nervous system, as evidenced by the occasional movements which most women feel during the later months of pregnancy. The liver, too, is building glucose and amino-acids into the substance of the body.

Variation

No two individuals, with the exception of identical twins derived from the same fertilized ovum, are, however, destined to grow up alike, and this mainly for genetic reasons. They have inherited different genes, as in the case of two of a different race, or within the same race they have inherited different configurations of the same genes. They are derived from different plans, and their development works out differently accordingly. Further, first on account of the crossing over of genes during the formation of the germ cells, and then on account of the random reconstitution of the chromosome pairs when an ovum is fertilized, the children of the same parents, identical twins excepted, are all derived from different plans, and destined to grow up different accordingly.

Variation may also be due to mutation, that is to say to alteration in the structure of a gene which leads it to exert a different effect on development in the future to that which it has exerted in the past. In insects this can be caused by exposing them to certain chemicals; in animals by submitting them to ionizing radiation. It also occurs spontaneously, certain mutations being more common than others. Most are disadvantageous, often so disadvantageous that they prove incompatible with life. Then pregnancy ends in abortion. Others are compatible with intra-uterine but incompatible with extra-uterine existence, and are bred out by premature death.

The origin of man

The mechanism which determines the inheritance of structure and function seems sufficiently rigid to perpetuate species in a world in which everything is tending to change. But it also seems to have been just sufficiently labile, and sufficiently subject to the influence of environment, to permit the necessary degree of variation for natural selection to work on in order to lead to organic evolution. Early in it, and in the case of the simpler forms of life evolving still, mutation figured, and figures, as the most important variety of genetic variation. It produced new cards, so to speak, with which the mechanism of heredity could play. Later mutation became less important, as the number of possible new mutations fell off, while the possibilities of the creation of new species by reshuffling of pre-existing cards, i.e. genes already existing, steadily increased.

The ordinary man, although he sees that natural selection must have operated, finds it difficult to conceive of chance mutation producing the cards and the formation of the germ cells and the re-combination of the chromosomes reshuffling them at random as *the* cause of the favourable variations on which it has worked to lead to organic evolution. But the time scale is vast, the number of genes and their possible permutations and combinations incalulable, and it is the opinion held by scientists today. On this view, the genetic plan for man was determined, like the genetic plan for all species that now exist or ever have existed, by that which is generally called chance.

Until recently chance would have been defined as the net result of complex interactions between innumerable combinations and permutations of minor cause and effect which were, on the one hand, so small, and, on the other, so numerous, that they defied analysis. For science was still dominated by the concept of relentless natural laws and the rigid sequence of cause and effect. Every event had a definite antecedent event to which it was due. It could not happen without it. So, granted the necessary knowledge, all happenings were predictable. Uncertainty was entirely on our part, and mainly due to ignorance, and in ordinary life chance is, of course, as above defined. But the rise of quantum mechanics has changed our outlook. At the sub-atomic level, a basic principle of uncertainty seems to be built into nature. If we possessed all knowledge, we still would not know which atom in a gram of radium was destined to break down next, and it seems likely that mutation and other events in molecular biology are also unpredictable in this sense. Whence it follows that, if all relevant facts had been available to mind existing when organic evolution started, both its course, and man, its highest product, could not have been predicted. Further, if it started again, it might take an entirely different course.

How life started is not known, but it demanded two varieties of nitrogen-containing compounds of carbon, the nucleotides and the amino-acids. For the former provide the reproductive mechanism of cells, while the latter permit the synthesis of protein on which growth depends. Somehow these had to be synthesized, and somehow, too, they had to come together, and this presumably happened at some point in the history of the earth when oxygen, nitrogen, carbon dioxide and water were exposed at a certain temperature to ionzing radiation. In this view the origin of life is also due to an accidental combination of circumstances. Again it could hardly have been foreseen, if mind had been there to foresee it.

Whether life exists in some other planet as well as on this earth must now be regarded as a serious problem. All the necessary elements for its genesis are to be found widely distributed throughout the universe, and it now seems probable that many other planets exist in which the physical conditions have been, must be, or will be, much the same as they are on earth. For the angular momentum of the stars can be ascertained, and while 3 per cent of them have a high one, 97 per cent, including the sun, have a low one. If however the angular momentum of its planets is added to that of the sun, the sun jumps up into the high angular momentum category, suggesting that the low angular momentum of many stars is due to the fact they they have lost momentum to planets circulating round them, just as our sun has lost momentum to the planets circulating round it. So, as in view of the vast number of stars, there must be a vast number of planets, the chances of the physical conditions pertaining on a few of them at least having been, being, or becoming right for the genesis and maintenance of life, particularly in view of the magnitude of astronomical time, must be very high indeed.

The last link in the argument for the existence of life elsewhere is, however, missing. We know that life did start on the earth, but we do not know what were the chances of it happening. Was it almost inevitable, or just chance? There is no answer to that question. But if life already exists, has existed, or one day will exist elsewhere, it does not follow that it is or will be life as we know it here.

*   *   *

The individual human body is the result of a plan laid at its conception when the germ cells of its parents fused, modified in the course of its execution by the environment in which that developed—just one case of the execution of the general human plan, the result of millions of years of the natural selection of fortuitous variations in the struggle for existence. Matter, energy, the elements, and the laws which govern their behaviour, started somehow, and then at a certain stage in the world's history, life whence all human life is derived, came into being, the conditions for the synthesis of the kind of matter on which it depends being at that moment favourable.

CHAPTER III

HORMONES AND THE
NERVOUS SYSTEM

*The endocrine organs—The nervous system—Muscle and
gland—Reflex action—Voluntary movement—Perception—
Consciousness—Sleep—Memory—The frontal lobes.*

Birth is a transient episode in a continuous process governed by
the genes. Growth, increase in size by cell division, and development, maturation of function, continue uninterrupted, the one
dependent on the other. But both depend secondarily on hormones secreted by the endocrine glands straight into the blood.
These have a profound effect on them, and, like all parts of the
body, come into action according to the plan laid at conception
and the inborn time schedule. Further, they play an active part
in promoting emotional states and regulating function in relation to need.

The endocrine organs

The most important of these hormone-secreting glands is the
pituitary situated at the base of the brain and connected to the
hypothalamus by a short stalk.

Four pituitary hormones exercise a direct action on function.
One regulates the growth in length and width of bone, and is
largely responsible for the height and general architecture of the
body. Another resists excessive loss of water, and helps to maintain that constant concentration of salt and other electrolytes in
our blood and systemic fluids which is essential to life. The
other two are important in relation to parturition and lactation.

Four others control the activity of other endocrine organs.
Thyrotropine regulates the secretion of thyroxine and, like the
hand throttle of a motor car, sets the level at which the machinery

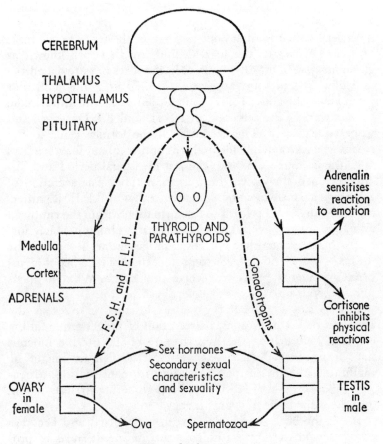

CEREBRUM

THALAMUS
HYPOTHALAMUS

PITUITARY

Adrenalin
sensitises
reaction
to emotion

Medulla

Cortex

ADRENALS

THYROID AND
PARATHYROIDS

F.S.H. and F.L.H.

Gonadotropins

Cortisone
inhibits
physical
reactions

Sex hormones
Secondary sexual
characteristics
and sexuality

OVARY
in
female

TESTIS
in
male

Ova   Spermatozoa

The endocrine system

of the body ticks over at rest. It is also responsible for the quality
of physical development. Without its help, a child grows up a
cretin, coarse in body and deficient in mind. The adreno-
corticotropic hormone (A.C.T.H.) regulates the secretion of
cortisone by the adrenal which protects the body against
physical stress, mechanical injury and exposure to cold. A third
is responsible for the regulation of the secretion of insulin which
enables the body to use sugar. A fourth regulates the secretion
of parathormone by the parathyroid glands. This mobilizes

calcium in the service of the growth and maintenance of bone. Further, at puberty the pituitary starts to secrete two separate hormones which both act on the gonads, the testes in the male and the ovaries in the female, and are therefore known as gonadotropic. They are identical in the sexes but are called the follicular stimulating hormone, F.S.H. and the follicular luteinizing hormone, F.L.H., after their action in the female.

In a woman the secretion of F.S.H. and F.L.H. waxes and wanes alternately. The secretion of the former leads to the ripening of a Graafian follicle which ruptures about fourteen days after the commencement of the last menstrual period and discharges an ovum down the Fallopian tube. The secretion of F.S.H. then starts to wane. Meanwhile that of F.L.H. is gathering strength, and this leads to the formation within the ruptured follicle of a mass of cells known as the corpus luteum which now starts to secrete another hormone, progesterone. Reaching the uterus by the blood, it leads to proliferation of its mucous membrane, getting it ready to receive that ovum. What happens next depends on whether it is fertilized or not.

If it is not fertilized, the corpus luteum regresses as the secretion of F.L.H. wanes, its secretion of progesterone falling off, and before long the hypertrophy of the uterine mucous membrane, for which it was responsible, can no longer be maintained. It breaks down, leading to menstruation. Meanwhile the secretion of F.S.H. has been gathering strength again, and the same cycle of events is repeated.

If, on the other hand, that ovum is fertilized and becomes embedded in the uterine mucous membrane, it starts to produce a hormone which, reaching the ovary by the blood, maintains the corpus luteum, and therefore progesterone secretion, in spite of the fact that the pituitary has stopped producing the F.L.H. on which it previously depended. So the proliferated and hypertrophied uterine mucous membrane, instead of breaking down, persists, and the fertilized ovum proceeds to develop under genetic control as described in the last chapter.

In a man F.S.H. and F.L.H. are both secreted more or less continuously. There is no cycle as in the female. Pituitary F.S.H. is however responsible for the continuous production of spermatozoa, and in both sexes F.L.H. leads the interstitial cells in the gonads to produce the sex hormones, testosterone in the male and oestrogen in the female. These lead to the development of the secondary sexual characteristics, and are in part responsible for sexuality.

In general each component of the endocrine system works on the feed-back principle. The pituitary, for example, is sensitive to thyroxine in the sense that if the level of it in the blood falls, the pituitary puts out more thyrotropic hormone. This increases the thyroid activity, and the thyroid puts out more thyroxine. But rise of thyroxine in the blood reduces the secretion of pituitary thyrotropine. Thyroxine level therefore falls again. In this way a constant concentration of thyroxine in the blood is maintained according to the level at which pituitary sensitivity to thyroxine is set.

The nervous system

Chemical control of function is relatively slow. Immediate response, when the necessity arises, is provided by the quick-acting nervous system.

The brain consists of a primitive stem (the upward extension of the spinal cord) and certain structures derived from it. The spinal cord consists of thirty-one more or less uniform segments. Peripheral nerves connect brain and spinal cord (the central nervous system) with all parts of the body. One set, called somatic or skeleto-sensory-motor, link it up with our skin and muscles; another, called autonomic or sympathetic, with our hearts, lungs, kidneys, intestinal tracts, sweat glands, salivary glands and endocrine glands. Microscopically the whole system is made up of neurones, each one a single cell with a number of short branches or dendrons, and one long fibre or axon. This latter may be up to two feet in length, and is covered by a white 'insulating' material. Every nerve fibre is developed from, and essentially part of, a nerve cell.

Nerve fibres conduct impulses. This depends on the fact that while some substances—sugar for instance—retain their molecular structure when they disappear in solution, others such as salts, acids and alkalies, dissociate completely or partly into ions. NaCl, for example, dissociates into a positively charged sodium ion and a negatively charged chlorine ion; potassium

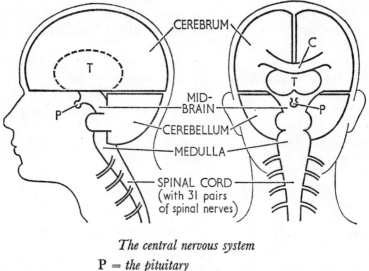

The central nervous system
P = *the pituitary*
T = *the thalamus*
C = *the corpus callosum*

chloride, KCl, into similarly charged potassium and chlorine ions; hydrochloric acid, HCl, into a positively charged hydrogen ion and a negatively charged chlorine ion. Even water is partially dissociated into positively charged H ions and negatively charged OH ions, of necessity equal in number.

Every cell contains sodium and potassium chloride in solution, and stimulation of a nerve fibre leads to a sudden redistribution of ions at that point with a corresponding alteration of electric potential. This travels rapidly down the fibre, its passage easily detected by means of electrodes, connected through a galvanometer, placed on it. Normally impulses are started by chemical or mechanical stimulation (we see chemically and hear mechanically). But in experimental work, electrical stimulation is more convenient as it can be graded, and by this means it has been shown that an impulse does not start until a certain threshold intensity of stimulation has been reached; also that, after an impulse has travelled down it, a nerve is incapable of conducting another until the *status quo* has been restored at the

38

expense of energy derived from its environment. All nerve impulses are of the same intensity. But, if the rate and strength of stimulation is increased, the number of impulses started per unit of time and the number of fibres carrying impulses are both increased, and it is the rate at which impulses arrive at their destination and the number of fibres involved which determine the rate of secretion by a gland and the force of contraction of a muscle.

All impulses are in fact qualitatively the same, the function of a sensory nerve, whether it is concerned with pain, temperature, touch or sight, depending, not on the nature of the impulse travelling in it, but on its connection in the cord or brain. Similarly, the function of a motor nerve, whether it is concerned with kicking, sneezing, or crying, depends again, not on the nature of the impulses travelling in it, but on the muscles it supplies. Fibres do not conduct sensation or carry orders. They transmit signals, and all these signals are qualitatively the same, the result of the arrival of an impulse depending, not on its nature, but on the set-up at that point. Just as the same make or break of constant current can blow up a ton of T.N.T., or merely turn a tap, so the arrival of a nerve impulse can, on the one hand, make a muscle contract, or stop it doing so, on the other.

There are ten billion neurones in the nervous system, interlacing with each other, and the question arises as to why an

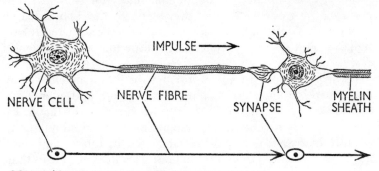

Neurones

impulse entering this complicated network does not immediately spread all over it, activating every structure supplied by it. The answer lies in the fact that axons and dendrons never quite touch, impulses being carried across the minute gaps between them by the rapid formation, and equally rapid destruction (as soon as their work is done), of specific chemical substances. The rate of this varies, and in consequence impulses do not 'jump' all synaptic junctions equally easily everywhere. Rather, paths of low resistance get laid down. Further, impulses can only cross synaptic junctions in one direction. Traffic is, in fact, one way, and neurones can be divided from the point of view of what they do into three groups: efferent or effector, afferent or receptor, and intermediate or connector. Efferent conduct impulses from the brain or cord to all parts of the body; afferent from the skin, muscles and internal structures to the cord or brain. Connector neurones link afferent and efferent neurones together within the nervous system, either directly or through networks of neurones of like kind.

Muscle and gland

There are two kinds of muscle which differ in appearance and in the function which they serve: striped or voluntary, and plain or involuntary.

Striped muscle, so-called because its fibres present a striated appearance under the microscope, is attached at both its ends to bone, and provides the motor machinery for changing our position, using our hands, and moving our bodies about. It has a single nerve supply, and in general only acts on receipt of signals from the nervous system. It is little under the influence of our emotions.

Unstriped or plain muscle provides the motor machinery of the gastro-intestinal tract, bile duct, ureters and uterus. A special variety of it in the heart helps to circulate the blood. In general it acts involuntarily, responding to local stimulation, notably increased tension—it is arranged in tubes—and does not need any signal to go into action. This does not mean that it has no nerve supply. As a matter of fact it has a double supply: one which increases, and the other which diminishes, its response to local stimulation. Further, plain muscle is under emotional rather than volitional control. A man cannot increase the rate at which his heart beats by taking thought, but it accelerates automatically during exercise and under emotional stress.

Glands, organs which manufacture substances vital to the economy of the body, are also of two kinds: those that secrete their products externally—like the glands in the wall of the stomach and the sweat glands in our skin—and those—like the thyroid and adrenal—which secrete them straight into our blood. Some, as a matter of fact, do both. The pancreas, for example, secretes a digestive juice into the gut and insulin into our blood. The gonads form the gametes, and secrete the sex hormones. While, however, some muscles are under our voluntary control, and have a single nerve supply, and others lie outside it, and have a double one, all glands fall into the latter category. All lie outside our voluntary control, and like plain muscle have a double nerve supply. One set increases and the other decreases their activity. This is much influenced by our emotions.

Reflex action

Organs are provided with sensory nerve fibres. These start in end-organs sensitive to touch, pain, heat or cold in our skin and mucous membranes, and in others sensitive to tension or position in our muscles, joints, gastro-intestinal tracts, hearts and arteries. All converge on the segment of the nervous system corresponding to that whence that particular organ or part of it is derived. For the body is segmental in origin. Twelve primitive segments in the region of the mouth fused to form the head, anatomical evidence for their one-time relative independence being afforded by the twelve pairs of nerves escaping from the skull. Thirty segments gave rise to the rest of the body. These can still be recognized in the vertebrae and in the pairs of nerves which pass out through the gaps between them.

In the cord and brain stem a complex network of fibres connects all incoming and outgoing neurones at and between all levels, and at all levels between both sides. An entering impulse would, as we have already seen, spread all over the nervous system, were not paths of low resistance which impulses tend to take gradually laid down. This is the basis of reflex action. Impulses coming from a certain point in the body always travel along the same path, and lead to the same result. Reflexes of this kind regulate both visceral and skeleto-motor function. Some of these paths are inherited. Others are acquired as the result of experience or practice.

Reflexes of which we are largely unaware adapt visceral function to the needs of the body in relation to changing situations. Exposure to cold, for example, leads, through a heat-regulating centre, to readjustment of heat production in relation to heat loss in such a way as to keep the temperature constant. Reflexes through a cardio-inhibitory centre control the rate of the heart, and through a vaso-motor centre, regulate the blood pressure. Reflexes through a respiratory centre, whose sensitivity to afferent stimuli from the lungs is determined by the acidity of the blood which depends on its content of carbon dioxide, regulate the rate and depth of breathing. Pulmonary ventilation is in fact geared to the requirement of the body in respect of the elimination of carbon dioxide, and normally this maintains an oxygen pressure in the lungs sufficient to saturate the arterial blood.

At the head and tail of the body, visceral reflexes play a daily part in the routine of living, and can be either facilitated or resisted by the action of muscles which are under our voluntary control. We can swallow more or less at will, although it is much easier to let it happen reflexively. Micturition, in response to rising intravesical tension, and defaecation, in response to filling of the rectum, can similarly be initiated, facilitated or resisted, by the action of voluntary muscles that can be brought into play at will. Other reflexes are protective, many of them depending on the action of voluntary muscle. Sneezing and coughing, for instance, which interrupt the normal rhythm of respiration because they use the same muscles, keep the airway clear. Vomiting, another reflex through a centre in the medulla, protects the stomach. Reflex flinching through the eyes protects them and the head from the coming blow. This reflex cannot be resisted, and this statement is also true of the reflex withdrawal of any part of the body which results from sudden painful stimulation.

In all reflex acts many, sometimes dozens, of muscles are

involved. When a man treads on something sharp, not only must the action of all his muscles in that leg be readjusted in such a way as to withdraw it, but his other leg must be quickly extended to take the weight of his body, while those of his trunk need to come into action in such a way as to tilt it, and preserve his balance—a feat of co-ordination only rendered possible by the fact that muscles are provided with receptor organs sensitive to tension and position. These give rise to impulses which, by virtue of the connections of the fibres in which they travel in the nervous system, keep it 'informed' of their state of contraction. When in fact any part of the body starts to move, thousands of impulses flood into the nervous system, but always result, in consequence of the way in which it has evolved, in all the muscles concerned doing just the right thing.

This computer mechanism of the nervous system, if we may venture to call it that, can go one better than any designed by man in that the neurone unit of the former is more efficient than the electronic unit of the latter. In order to make man-designed computer do something new, it is necessary to take it down and re-wire it. But the human computer is provided with an ample supply of spare neurones, and can learn by experience, a fact which depends on a property of synaptic junctions already pointed out. The repeated transmission of impulses across them lowers resistance at them with the result that paths of low resistance are established. This is the physiological basis of learning. In addition to *inheriting* paths of low resistance which underlie our protective reflexes, we *learn*, as we grow up, to balance and walk, and then to play games, catch and hit balls. This involves accepting and rejecting vast numbers of entering impulses from our eyes and muscles, recording and storing them, calling on them when required, in short processing a vast quantity of incoming information at speed so as to give the necessary directions to our muscles immediately.

Many inherited reflexes and many of those acquired during life, enabling us to perform acts of great complexity without conscious thought, demand the use of the same muscles in different ways, and cannot be performed together. It is impossible to swallow *and* breathe; impossible to breathe *and* strain; impossible to run *and* jump. Again and again the nervous

43

system takes a decision, and we know from our own experience how, at a certain point, we stop breathing to swallow, or stop straining to breathe, or stop walking to jump. The situation at length compels a choice, and this appears to be determined by the reticulo-activating system, a mass of nerve cells which starts in the brain stem and extends upwards into the thalamic and hypothalamic regions. All the main channels of communication between the cord and cortex send collaterals into it in passing, and in this way it is kept 'informed' as to all signals travelling up the brain stem, while on the motor side it links up with every segment in the spinal cord, with the visceral centres in the brain stem, and with the cerebral cortex on both sides.

The reticulo-activating system, ranging wide in this way, can also enhance or diminish nervous action arising from other sources. In short, to use a sound analogy, it seems to act as a sort of volume control in respect of a recording already turned on. Signals are sent down its effector fibres, and these form synaptic junctions with the same motor nerve cells as those which send their fibres to the muscles, the lower motor neurones, which execute orders issued by the cortex. (See next section.) This action may be motor or inhibitor, and the latter may be so strong that it calls these orders off, and lets a different set into the final common path, completely altering the pattern of response when a situation urgently demands it.

Further, in the hypothalamus this system appears to control the pituitary gland which, as we have already seen, regulates the activity of all the other endocrine glands. Here the arrival of signals relating to the state of the body 'decides', by means of some sort of computer machinery, whether in the light of the situation prevailing any alteration in the relative secretion of these glands is required. For one situation, for example, a sexual one, clearly requires different endocrine adjustments to a situation associated with hiding, fighting, or running away. Just in fact as patterns of reflex action are stored in the cord, so patterns of endocrine secretion are stored in the hypothalamus. In short the reticulo-activating system provides the connecting link between the two main mechanisms of bodily control: our quick acting trigger-pulling nervous system, on the one hand, and our slow acting reinforcing hormonal system on the other.

Voluntary movement

The determination to resist a reflex and the idea of executing a movement are vested in what a man rather vaguely calls his mind. Its orders are executed at the physiological level.

Stimulation of a certain area of the cerebral cortex, the motor area, always leads to movement of the same part of the body on the opposite side; the upper part of it always to movement of the leg; the lower part of it, always to movement of the arm, hand or face. Whence we infer that when a man wills the movement of any part of his right side, cells in his left cortex initiate impulses which travel down his brain stem, cross to the opposite side, and end by forming synaptic junctions with the cells in the cord which send their effector fibres direct to the skeletal muscles. These fibres constitute the path which all impulses must take to reach the muscles, the final common path, and they can be got at in two ways: reflexively or voluntarily. In other words, the same movement can be reflex or voluntary, and much of our apparent voluntary movement—for example, walking—depends on the cortex triggering off patterns of reflex action already latent in the cord. This is economic. The cerebral cortex is free to concentrate on movements seldom performed normally.

Voluntary movement also demands co-ordination. Without some mechanism to promote it, playing the piano or returning a service at tennis would be impossible, and it would be idle to pretend that we know how things like those are done. But we are aware of two mechanisms which clearly play some part. In the first place, impulses from receptors deep in our muscles and joints are always arriving in the cortex just behind the motor area. We do not look to see where our arms and legs are in order to realize their position in space. These keep us aware of it. In the second, impulses which do not impinge on consciousness are always arriving in the cerebellum which also receives signals from the semi-circular canals in the internal ear. These latter contain receptors sensitive to change of pressure caused by movement of the fluid in them because of rotation of the body or alteration of its position. The cerebellum is in fact largely responsible for the co-ordination of movement of all kinds. It

45

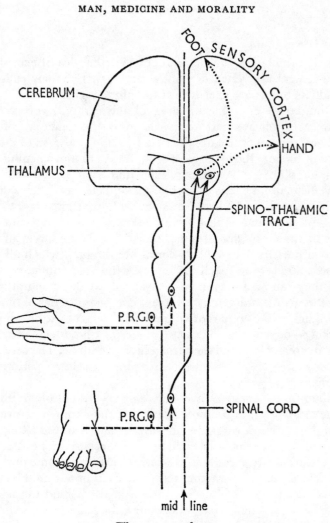

The motor pathways

acts, to adopt an analogy from engineering, as a stabilizer, maintaining our balace when we ride a bicycle, play tennis, or perform any movement in which the whole body is involved.

Perception

Skin, mucous membrane and muscle are provided with special

46

end organs which lower the threshold to one special form of stimulation, and raise it to all others, with the result that every peripheral nerve is always carrying a collection of impulses underlying touch, temperature, position, and sometimes pain, into the segment of the spinal cord corresponding to that of the body whence that skin, mucous membrane and muscle were derived. Here they form synaptic junctions with cells giving rise to a second lot of neurones, and, in the hand-over, impulses are classified according to function. All impulses underlying touch, all underlying temperature, all underlying position, all underlying pain, now travel up in bundles together, cross the middle line, and end in the thalamus, a collection of nerve cells lying deep between the two cerebral hemispheres. Here these signals are converted into composite consciousness of touch, temperature, position and pain of a crude kind. A third set of fibres relay them to an area in the cerebral cortex just behind the motor area, and here they are transposed into consciousness accurately. It is in the cortex that we become aware, for instance, of the exact size, shape, weight, texture and exact temperature of an object grasped in the hand and, if it has sharp edges, painfully aware of them. We say we feel it in our hand. As a matter of fact we feel it in the cortex, and refer all sensation associated with it to our hand.

The lens of the eye throws an inverted image of that on which it is focused on to the retina. There the impact of light of different wave-lengths leads to the immediate synthesis of chemical substances, which in turn start impulses, which in turn transmit signals (again all qualitatively the same, and differing only in the point whence they come) to the visual cortex in the occipital lobes. Again, too, we meet the same phenomenon of crossing over, impulses from the left side of the left retina being conveyed to the right occipital cortex. Here, too, these signals are transposed into consciousness, the way in which a man sees his immediate environment depending in part on his mechanism for doing it. He may be colour blind, for instance. A cat, too, sees the world very differently to a man; a frog, we believe, differently to a cat.

The ear dissects sound for transmission just as the eye dissects light. In the ear a series of receptors vibrate to different

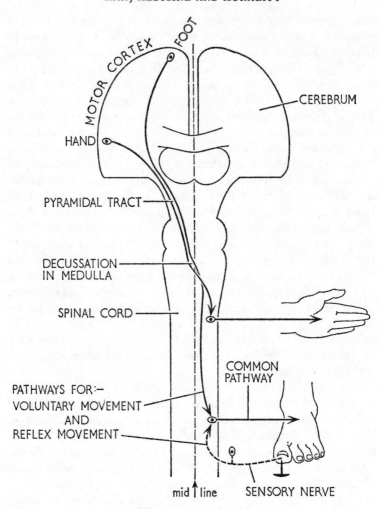

The sensory pathways
P.R.G. = *posterior root ganglion*

frequencies, each one starting signals which are conveyed in the fibres of the auditory nerves to the cortex of the temporal lobes where they are resynthesized into the sound pictures which gave rise to them.

Smell, although important in the life of animals, plays little

48

part in that of man, but it is one of the most accurate senses, and depends on individual nerve endings being sensitive to stimulation by certain chemical substances. The same principle holds. A composite smell is dissected into its component parts by nerve endings in the nasal mucous membrane, and signals sent accordingly to the cerebral cortex at the base of the brain on the opposite side. Again these are all qualitatively the same, differing only in the point whence they come. Here, as in the case of sight and hearing, the cortex reconstructs the total smell, and transposes it into consciousness.

The sensory is in fact constructed like the motor nervous system, and also like much of the rest of the body, in two symmetrical halves, with cortical sensory areas, duplicated on the two sides. It might have been thought that the result would be a left-handed mind and a right-handed mind, the left not knowing what the right was doing. This has been provided against. At all levels bundles of fibres connect the corresponding sensory areas on the two sides. The largest of these, the corpus callosum, connects visual area with visual area, auditory area with auditory area, the sensory area on one side with the sensory area on the other.

We are conscious of the environment in which we live, it can therefore be said, because we are armed with receptors specifically sensitive to different aspects of it. We are not endowed with the necessary receptors to detect everything that is going on in and round about us. We are not conscious of the atmosphere, for example, except when it moves, and we call it wind, or when the pressure of it falls as we go up a mountain, and our ears pop; of X-rays passing through our bodies or of cosmic rays in our atmosphere. Nevertheless, we are well provided with them, and able to form what we believe to be a more or less true picture of our environment, and of the relation of our bodies to it, in terms of shape, weight, movement, colour, smell and sound. Further, not only are we conscious of living in three-dimensional space, but also aware of the passage of time, although how we appreciate it is not yet understood.

Perception is more complex than might have been supposed however. A man who has been born blind, but recovers his sight in later life, does not immediately see the world like one who has been blessed with normal vision from the start. He has to learn to see, and cases are recorded of men in this situation who have found the task so difficult that they have never succeeded. For perception does not merely depend on the sensory information arriving at the moment, but on its integration in the light of past experience. We learn how to percieve, as we grow up, and some are better at doing it than others.

To what extent we can ever know what the real world is like is a difficult question. Up to a certain point, and in certain respects, we clearly do know it. Unless we take the necessary steps to avoid the solid object we see, we fall over it, and, if we ignore time, we are caught by nightfall or miss our train. In short, we can be certain of the real existence, apart from ourselves, of time and space in three dimensions. But is the grass really green, and does the brook really babble except in the perception of the man who hears it? Physical science replies that the grass is only green because it absorbs all the light in the spectrum, except the green, and that, reflected from it and falling on a man's retina, leads to a succession of physical events in his nervous system which results in him being conscious of green. According to physical science we dress up the real world of space-time in colour and sound, and different men and animals see and hear it differently according to the machinery of perception with which they are endowed. A frog sees moving spots. Some birds possess a greater range of colour vision than man. Some men are colour blind. But there can be no satisfying answers to questions of this kind. For the mind of man is a component of the experience which it so much wants to explain. He is not a detached observer. Rather, he is part of the universe which he is trying to observe.

Consciousness

Perception demands consciousness, and this does not depend on the cerebral cortex alone. It also depends in part on a centre in the reticulo-activating system in the upper brain stem sending impulses up to all parts of the cerebral cortex, sensitizing it to incoming stimuli, pepping it up and keeping it on its job. Further, it is now known that all neurones carrying impulses underlying potential conscious sensation to the cortex send collateral branches into it, pepping it up in anticipation of their own arrival. And this pepped-up state of the cortex can be demonstrated. If electrodes are placed on a man's head and connected through a galvanometer, rapid irregular waves of low potential, the so-called α rhythm, are recorded when he is fully awake and alert, and lying quietly with his eyes closed. These do not indicate thoughts or perceptions. Indeed, they disappear if he opens his eyes, is shouted at, or given a problem to solve. Rather, they indicate general cortical activity initiated by the reticulo-activating system, a brain in a state of readiness to attend to any stimuli which may come along. It is on this state that consciousness depends. If the cortex is cut off from the brain stem, so that impulses cannot get to it from the reticulo-activating system, a man lapses into an unconscious state and the α rhythm of wakefulness gives way to slow irregular high voltage waves identical with those recorded in natural sleep. Animal experiments have also shown that centres of different

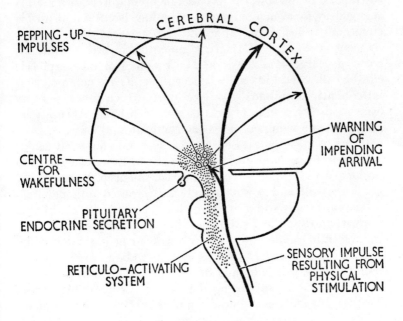

The mechanism of keeping awake

kinds exist in the reticulo-activating system associated with emotional feeling. Stimulation of a centre in it in one way destroys appetite; in another way increases it out of all proportion to need. Stimulation of centres in the hypothalamic region of monkeys produces rage or fear, while stimulation of others leads to transitory pleasure or to pain. At first it was thought that the rage, fear, pain or pleasure were artificial, that the animal was merely exhibiting the physical concomitants of the emotion without actually experiencing it. But experiments permitting the animal a choice have shown that the emotion is really felt. The animal must actually experience the pleasure or the punishment because it presses the lever, which it has learnt to work, again and again, either to get what it likes or to avoid what it so dislikes. These centres are fundamental to animal nature. Basic desires are satisfied by stimulation of them.

Sleep

As the day draws towards its close, or prematurely, if a man is engaged in some monotonous occupation, his attention to his environment begins to lapse, and he starts to doze. As this happens, the waves of electric potential recorded from his cortex get larger and slower, and in this phase of half-sleep, as it can be called, odd ideas and queer thoughts are common, not infrequently terminated by sleep starts which are sometimes associated with a flash of light or a sudden bang. Abruptly he returns to consciousness of his environment, and endeavours to get back to grips with it but, often as not, soon dozes off again.

Eventually, after any long period of being awake, he falls into prolonged sleep. The waves on his electro-encephalogram now get slower still, and he is no longer easily aroused, although he is woken up by any stimulus to which he is peculiarly sensitive; a mother, for example, by the cry of her child while the noise of a passing train remains unheard. At this stage he is not dreaming, and his muscles are not relaxed, but after about an hour and a half he begins to dream, and this is associated with rapid movement of the eyes, suggesting that he is looking at his dream. Further, his muscles are now completely relaxed. Many maintain that they never dream, but waking people up and asking them reveals that everyone does. Most dreams are in fact forgotten. The non-dreamer is a man who habitually forgets his dreams.

There are in fact two kinds of sleep: that with large waves on the E.E.G. and contracted muscles, without dreams; and that with small waves and completely relaxed muscles, with dreams. The former, when first discovered, was regarded, in view of the complete unconsciousness associated with it, as deep sleep; the latter, in view of its association with dreams, as light sleep. But partially contracted muscles are inconsistent with the concept of deep sleep; completely relaxed muscles inconsistent with that of light sleep. Besides, it is as difficult to rouse a man out of one kind of sleep as it is to rouse him out of the other. The difference between these two known forms of sleep is not related to depth. They are now known instead as orthodox and paradoxical sleep respectively.

These varieties of sleep alternate in periods of about one and a half hours each in a normal man throughout the night, but if he has been deprived to sleep for a long period, orthodox sleep persists throughout the greater part of his first night of renewed normal sleep. Next night far more time is spent in paradoxical than in orthodox sleep. He is catching up, as it were, on the paradoxical sleep he missed the night before which suggests that both kinds of sleep serve a purpose; orthodox sleep the needs of the body, paradoxical sleep, perhaps, those of the mind developed on it. Indeed, it has been suggested that the dream formation which goes with the latter is as necessary to the health of the mind as getting rid of the waste products of metabolism is necessary to the health of the body.

This hypothesis provides a possible *raison d'être* for the strange phenomenon of dreaming, and some of our dreams are clearly related to our conscious hopes, fears, and worries. To some extent, too, they are related to our environment. Spray a sleeping man with water, and he may dream that he has been caught in the rain. Most dreams, however, are completely incomprehensible to us, but represent, according to Freudian theory, unconscious wish-fulfilment in relation to instinct camouflaged in the symbolism of primitive ways of thought. Alternatively, although all dreams are clearly capable of psychoanalytical interpretation, most of them—and we remember only a very small proportion of them—may well be due to the mind working at random uncontrolled by environment or will.

Memory

We forget our dreams but we remember events in our lives, and the recent psychological approach to the study of the mind shows that we store far more of our experience in memory than our powers of recall would lead us to suppose.

Stimulation of the cortex of the temporal lobe *occasionally* forces some aspect of past experience back into consciousness. These are true memories of events, that is to say, recollections of things known to have happened. They never partake of the nature of delusions or hallucinations but, contrary to what might have been expected, are invariably of an inconsequential kind. There never seems any good reason why that particular experience should have been resurrected, and they are experiences which are not ordinarily recalled. Rather, they are of the kind thought forgotten, experience deemed 'gone for good'. Nevertheless, they can be vivid, and the patient looks upon the recollection, not so much as sudden memory recall, but as actually living through that experience again, feeling for the moment as if he was possessed of double consciousness; on the one hand, aware of events going on around him; on the other, living in and through an experience of the past. The recollection runs its course, like a film turned on, as long as the stimulus is kept applied. When that is withdrawn, it stops. Then, if the stimulus is re-applied, it starts again where it left off. Further, it is sometimes possible to 'play' the same recollection over and over again by repeated stimulation of the same cortical area.

Memories of this kind can only be evoked by stimulation of the temporal lobe, suggesting that memory was located in it, but investigation has failed to confirm this hope of a quick answer to a baffling problem. Destruction of one temporal lobe in man, and experimental removal in monkeys, does not lead to any appreciable loss of memory. Further, it is little affected when the frontal lobes are extensively damaged, and a cat or dog which has had all connections between frontal cortex and brain stem divided is still capable of learning and remembering simple tasks. In short, we do not know how we remember. On the other hand, in view of the way in which the mind seems to work, there is a high probability that memory depends on neurone circuits of some kind. Every now and then we forget something, a name or a word, and then, when we stop trying to recall it, sooner or later it flashes into consciousness again.

The frontal lobes

The motor area is the departure platform for impulses under-lying movement; the area immediately behind it, the arrival platform for those underlying sensation; and, as has just been seen, stimulation of the temporal lobe occasionally initiates the recall of a lost memory. But these areas comprise less than a quarter of the total surface of the cortex. All the rest is silent in the sense that stimulation of it never leads either to conscious sensation or to muscular action.

Most of this silent cortex is frontal, and the frontal lobes are larger in man and the apes than in any other animals, and better developed in the higher monkeys than in any of the rest. Further, there appears to be a definite correlation between frontal lobe development and intellectual capacity. So our frontal lobes have long been held responsible for the physio-logical processes underlying intellectual activity. Further, des-truction of a small area, Broca's area, in the dominant one—the left in a right-handed person—leads to aphasia, that is to say, inability to find the right words to express thoughts. Localiza-tion of speech is far from absolute however. Subsidiary centres exist, and different centres for the various aspects of it, finding words and letters, recognizing them in reading, stringing them together into sentences, have never been demonstrated.

Disease affecting other parts of the frontal lobes in man, and experimental ablation of them in monkeys, leads to much less serious consequences than was at one time expected, as exempli-fied by the case of Phineas Gage, a foreman in a road construc-tion gang. As the result of a mishap an iron rod passed through his skull, severely damaging his left frontal lobe and to some extent his right. Before the accident he is said to have been 'hard-working and shrewd, efficient and well balanced in his outlook on life'. Immediately after it he lay unconscious for an hour, and then managed to walk to see a surgeon, 'talking with

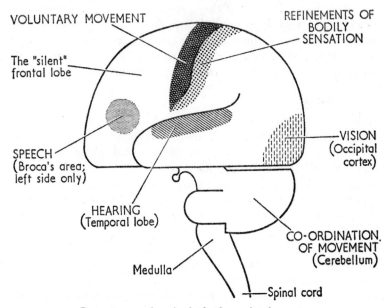

Departure and arrival platforms in the cortex

composure and equanimity of the hole in his head'. He subsequently developed a severe infection, but recovered and lived twelve years more but became, it is said, 'irreverent, profane and impatient of restraint, obstinate, yet capricious and vacillating'. Further, he now showed little consideration for others, and seemed intellectually simple but exhibited little loss of memory. He never worked again, and became a vagrant, scraping a living by showing himself off and telling his story.*

The traditional belief in the importance of the frontal lobes could no longer be upheld, and this conclusion has been confirmed by the brain injuries of two world wars, modern cerebral surgery, and experiments on apes.

In so far as generalization is possible, frontal lobe damage seems to lead to verbal impoverishment. Patients continue to speak grammatically, if Broca's area escapes, but they have difficulty in finding any great number of words in which to ex-

* Harlow, J. M. 1868. *Recovery after severe injury to the Head.* Publications Mass. Med. Soc. II, 329.

press their thoughts, and in consequence talk little. Past memories and skills are not lost, and intelligence tests before and after show little change, but they do have difficulty in dealing simultaneously with many concepts and forming judgments on abstract situations. The most common consequence of it is alteration in personality. A man who has been ambitious, well adjusted, highly motivated and considerate, now often comes to exhibit lack of drive, insensitivity to the feelings of others, diminished initiative, tactlessness, selfish behaviour and lack of appreciation of ethical and moral situations. He may become euphoric, that is to say, unduly elated, or restless, perpetually roaming about without any of the imaginative thinking which would be expected with it. A few lose emotional control, and get attacks of inordinate laughter or fly into tempers without apparent cause. Leucotomy, too (p. 176), although often successful for the purpose for which it was intended, is often only performed at the expense of some deterioration in personality. The results of cerebral damage are in fact variable, but nearly always far greater in a highly-developed, well-educated, sensitive person than in an average man, and in children it seems to have distastrous effect on personality development. Therefore we are driven to conclude that, just as the refinements of movement are latent in the motor cortex, and those of perception in the sensory cortex, so the refinements of the higher faculties of mind are vested in the silent areas of the frontal lobes.

*   *   *

To what extent can we claim to understand how the nervous system works in maintaining that which man calls his mind?

We do know the arrival platforms of impulses underlying different forms of sensation and the departure ones for those underlying voluntary movement. We also know that the brain is constructed, like the rest of the body, in two symmetrical halves with sensory areas and motor areas duplicated on its two sides, in spite of which the left hand does know what the right is doing, and we feel ourselves to be one person. Further, vital functions, instinct, pleasure, pain and emotion are centred in the brain stem. But recent work on the frontal lobes has revealed their surprising unimportance in relation to mental processes hitherto attributed to them, and this has largely sunk the view, until recently held, that certain higher centres ran the brain in relation to the mind. Rather, more in accordance with modern modes of thought is the recent concept that the brain works as an organic whole in maintaining the mind; that it is in fact in this respect a self-maintaining, although essentially unstable, self-regulating machine, the supreme achievement to date, it can be claimed, of organic evolution.

But, although we can now describe the processing of incoming information up to a point in terms of computer engineering in relation to the co-ordination of movement and sensation and, if we did know where or how memory was stored, could perhaps *describe* how we find the right words and letters to express our thoughts in speech and writing, we know nothing yet about the physiology of the brain in terms of which we can *describe* conceptual thinking, still less *describe* moral sense, aesthetic appreciation or spiritual vision. And the word 'describe' is used deliberately. For, although it seems likely that all mental processes have physical concomitants, it is as meaningless to try to *explain* mental processes in physical terms as it would be to try to *explain* physical processes in terms of conscious experience. We can influence mental process either by physical action on the brain or by psychological action on the mind. But physiology can never *explain* the mind in the kind of terms that man would like it explained, although, as we get to know more about the brain, we shall no doubt be able to influence mental process by physical means even further than we can at present. Indeed, even if neurophysiology eventually succeeds in *describing* how we think, and neuropsychology enables us to see why we sometimes think straight and at other times crooked, our conscious experience of thinking, and the results of it, will still remain to be explained, if they ever are explained, in terms of concepts which the mind of man can form as the result of his experience of living.

CHAPTER IV

BODY-MIND

Genetics—Consciousness—Psychosomatic development—The embryology of personality—Childhood—Adolescence.

The body in general, and the brain, which relies on many of the functions of it, in particular, permits the development of that which man calls his mind. The evidence is overwhelming. Failure of the development of the brain is incompatible with that of the mind. Oxygen lack, vitamin deficiency, dehydration, lack of sugar in the blood, drugs, all have a profound effect on it, while organic disease, if it affects the brain or any function of the body on which the brain depends, leads to mental disorder. Further, mental characteristics are inherited, and it is impossible to conceive of that in any other way except through the body on which the mind is developed.

Genetics

Every infant inherits the urges associated with self-preservation, and the patterns of behaviour and emotional reaction which derive from them. It also inherits the capacity to develop certain specifically human capacities, the ability to learn to talk, read and write, and thereby to acquire, store and use knowledge; and also, to varying degrees, the ability to think originally and creatively, and to invent and plan ahead. Thirdly, it inherits some of the mental characteristics of its parents and near relatives, in the same way as it inherits some of their physical attributes.

Every infant is also destined to develop mental characteristics peculiarly its own. Just as it can differ for genetic reasons from its brothers and sisters in many of its physical characteristics, so it can differ for genetic reasons from them in many of its mental characteristics. And this for the same reason: the segregation of genes in the formation of the germ cells and their random

59

recombination at conception. Nor can mutation be ruled out in the genesis of a child which is exceptional in any direction in a way which cannot be explained in terms of heredity or the environment in which it was brought up.

In short, just as at conception a plan—which may be faulty in some minor or major respect—can be said to be laid which will condition the development of a body, so at the same moment a plan—which again may be faulty in some minor or major respect—can be said to be laid which will condition the development of a mind. Or, as it would be more correct to say, at conception a plan is laid which will condition the development of body-mind under the stimulus of experience. For body and mind, although we tend to think about them as separate, are, in certain respects at any rate, one and undivided. The genetic plan first conditions the development of the body, and then the body conditions the development of the mind, ensuring that the child develops all the ordinary human instincts. No new unit of human life can escape them. It also ensures that it is born predisposed to develop some of the characteristics of its progenitors. No new unit of human life can escape that either. It also ensures that it is born with a predisposition to develop certain characteristics peculiarly its own. Further, the genetic plan ties its mental development. Just as the plan in respect of the body determines whether a man *can* in due course become a good performer, say in some branch of athletics, so the plan for the brain determines whether a man *can* in due course become first-class in some attribute of mind, or must of necessity, however good his education, ever remain in that respect dull-witted.*

Consciousness

The development of the mind demands consciousness. This, the

* It is important to understand the word *conditioned* as used in this context. It is not the same as 'determined by', and perhaps an analogy will make its meaning clear. The surface of a blackboard and the curvature of a mirror *condition* the appearance of a man's writing on or his reflection in it respectively. Different surfaces can make the same handwriting look different. Different mirrors can make a man look all sorts of shapes. Conversely, two different blackboards could make two different handwritings look alike. Similarly two different curved mirrors can make a tall and short man both look the same height.

supreme mystery, cannot be defined. But everyone knows what it is like, and is familiar with his own degrees of it, losing it in sleep and regaining it when he wakes. Further, it would now appear to depend on activity in the reticulo-activating system (p. 44). This in turn depends on adequate oxygen and glucose supply, as determined by the co-operative action of many functions of the body.

When this is in action the millions of signals arriving every second in a man's sensory cortex—a neurone can conduct about ten a second—are synthesized into awareness of the particular corner of his environment at which he happens to be looking: of the sounds coming and smell emanating from it; of his contact with it through his senses of position, touch, temperature and pain. Further, he is conscious of his own body occupying space in it, and also of himself as a unit of life existing in it and in time.

When a man is conscious he can will his muscles into action through the departure platforms of impulses underlying voluntary movement in his motor cortex. He can also endeavour to suppress reflex action and the urge of instinct. In short, by virtue of being conscious, he feels endowed with the power of choice, and this fact, more than any other, leads him to a dual concept of his nature: spirit imprisoned within the bonds of human flesh.

When a man is conscious, he can, by virtue of his thalamus and sensory cortex, enjoy eating, drinking, sex; and suffer pain, cold, hunger and disappointment. In short, the fulfilment of instinct is pleasurable, and dictates behaviour, in consequence of which individuals and species both tend to survive, life in its crudest form being devoted to getting pleasure by satisfying instinct. An animal eats because it enjoys it, and reproduces for the same reason. Consciousness, too, permits emotional feeling, that which moves us (hence the derivation of the word), and emotional feeling not only increases physical pleasure and physical pain, but also reinforces action deriving from them. It determines how hard a man fights, how intensely he loves, and how desperately he endeavours to escape.

In man emotional feeling is complicated by the anticipation of what may happen or what the consequences of an act may be as the result of his ability to reason, to remember, and to learn by experience. Further, his interest may conflict with the happiness of someone else, from whom he gains emotional satisfaction in return, or with the welfare of society on which he himself is dependent for his own security. Love, which engenders emotion, leads to ambition, selfishness and jealousy, and these in their turn tend to breed rivalry and aggressiveness. Emotional satisfaction, too, is self-destructive. It breeds insecurity for the simple reason that the more a man possesses, the more he stands to lose. Is it better to possess nothing? Human optimism comes down against this view. 'Better to have loved and lost, than never to have loved at all'. Absolute happiness, short of religious conviction—God cannot disappear unless faith fails— is like perfect health, an unrealisable ideal. All that a man can do is to strive to gain maximum emotional satisfaction at minimum emotional cost.

When a man is conscious he can set himself a problem, start to think it out, and arrive at an answer. This requires an effort of will and an expenditure of mental energy. But he has little idea as to how he does it. For the brain works, as we have seen, in some respects like a vast computer. We recall out of memory, find words to express our thoughts and letters in which to write them down, and also form many other associations, without being any more aware of how we do it than we are of how we co-ordinate our muscles in effecting our movements. Just in fact as a man can use a car to get himself from place to place without possessing any idea as to how it works, so he can turn on his brain to recollect or associate without any idea as to how that works either. And the analogy can be carried further. Just as some people possess better cars than others, and there are bigger computers than others, so some people possess better cerebral machinery than others with which to do their mental work. These do it quicker, more correctly, and can tackle more complicated problems.

The actual stage of consciousness is small. It is impossible to look at two things, experience two emotions, solve two problems, at the same time. All the mind can do is to oscillate backwards and forwards between them, as when hope alternates with fear. Sometimes, too, it is so concentrated on some external experience, on some memory resurrected from the past, or on some immediate problem, that it cannot think of anything else. Or, it is so dominated by pain or pleasure, by fear that something will happen, or by the hope that something else will not, that it cannot concentrate on what it ought to be doing. The stream of conscious life is in fact made up of an endless succession of shifting scenes, only interrupted by sleep, and even that is often disturbed by dreams, partly determined by external events and partly by the random upsurge of instinct and associations from within.

But behind the shifting scenes of consciousness lies a vast store of memories, some important, others trivial, some emotional, others commonplace, some easily recalled, others thought forgotten. And this is no mere passive respository of past experience. In it hope and fear go round and round, uncensored thoughts persist, duty and desire conflict. Further, it is a man's subconscious which determines his unthought-out reactions which contribute so largely to his personality. Indeed, he is not, as he is apt to think, his conscious self, which goes to sleep and dreams, with a well-ordered store of memories at his beck and call. Rather, just as an iceberg is mainly under the water, so a man's mind is mainly subconscious, and his subconscious largely determines those habitual reactions to experience which add up to create his personality. But the conscious part of the mind is peculiarly important. For it is in it alone that what we call and feel to be the will operates, and it is the will alone which can reject the reactions of the subconscious which have been built up as the result of emotional reactions in infancy and early childhood.

Psychosomatic development

Few remember anything before the age of three, but psychoanalysis often reveals very early experiences of an emotional kind: hunger and its frustration and satisfaction, and an infant's awareness of its special relation to its mother; early memories of comfort and discomfort associated with the rhythmic working of its body. These, it is true, cannot ever be confirmed, and in the interpretation by one person of the subjective experience of another there is always the risk of turning on the interpretation

63

most expected. But the findings of them add up to create probability, and these memories of infancy reveal a primitive way of thinking only met in early childhood. Certainly at birth it looks as if an infant suddenly becomes conscious. It yells, as if in pain, and, once fed, looks happy and content. So, although behaviour is an uncertain guide to consciousness—a man under an anaesthetic may struggle as if in pain—there is little reason to doubt that an infant becomes conscious in a primitive kind of way when or soon after it is born.

The stage is now set, and a mind develops under the stimulus of experience, conditioned by the body. This ensures, as has been seen, the development of instinct; favours that of family and individual traits; and also sets a limit to the extent to which the mind *can*, as opposed to the extent to which it *does*, develop. Further, not only does the body condition the development of the mind, habitual reactions so developed interacting to create personality, but these reactions seem to react back on and influence the further development of the body with the result that character becomes written in the face and states of mind in the expression. Instead, therefore, of talking about body *and* mind, as if they were separate and distinct, like a rider and his horse (the one able to part company with the other), it is nearer the truths, as already foreshadowed, to think in terms of body *hyphen* mind.

We cannot, however, analyse the development of the mind in the same ways as it is possible to analyse a physical interaction. The gap between our understanding of body and our understanding of mind remains. When, for example, a man is afraid, due to stimulation of his centre for fear by memory, anticipation or a situation, we have no method of partitioning responsibility for his fear between the physical sensitivity of his centre and the intensity of the conscious stimulus. The same dangerous situation can have a different effect on two people, not only on account of their differing previous experience, but also on account of the relative sensitivities of their centres. The latter depend on the way they are made and on the level of hormone secretion at the time. These we cannot evaluate, although they must influence their reactions in much the same way that the level at which the sound control is set influences the playing of a record.

64

Psychosomatic development can in fact be studied at present only from the angle of subjective experience, i.e. psychological factors, and as yet only to a very limited extent from the angle of the conditioning process in the nervous system, i.e. somatic factors. And yet the latter, the physical sensitivity of the emotional centres in it and the action of hormones on them, must influence individual development profoundly. Our interpretation of psychosomatic development remains inevitably one-sided.

The embryology of personality

The foundations of the body are laid within the first six weeks from conception, and those of personality and conscience, it now seems certain, within the first few years from birth. Further, just as normal development of the body depends on each organ starting to develop in time, and not precociously or out of step with the rest, so normal development of personality depends on each potentiality starting to develop in time and not developing precociously or crowding out or keeping another back. While, however, the genetic plan in respect of the body is executed *in utero*, its execution in respect of the mind only starts at birth. The conditions for the former are standard. Those for the latter differ with the circumstances of childhood.

Infants are born conscious of pleasure and pain. They are also capable of emotional feeling, which intensifies their reactions. They are also endowed with genetic capacities which come into action according to the inborn time schedule as the development of the nervous system proceeds. Environment, on the other hand, has a profound effect on the relative development of these inborn potentialities, and thereby on the digestion of experience and the building of it up into the structure of personality. But the environment of childhood and the way in which an infant is handled both vary widely, the new-born being the innocent victim of its circumstances. It may be legitimate or illegitimate, wanted or unwanted, foundling or orphan, a first child, an only child, or the last of a large family; one of a fond but foolish mother and of an interested or disinterested father, of two parents living happily together, or two at loggerheads with one another and so, before long, the relict of a broken home.

E   65

When an infant is not sleeping, which is what it does most of the time at first, that being the nearest to its previous existence it can get, it clings to its mother. It apparently feels, if its mental state is to be inferred from its behaviour, conscious of its dependence on her in the strange world into which it has been abruptly born. For impulses arriving in its thalami now lead to pleasure and to discomfort of a primitive kind. The former derives from breast feeding, from the relief of visceral tension, and before long from movement, as it lies kicking in its cot. Discontent may be due to hunger, to cold—on account of its relatively large surface area it loses heat very quickly—to the nappy overdue for changing, or to an uncomfortable position in its cot. And its emotional centres in its brain stem are already active. Pleasure is reflected in a smile; discontent in anger, as it struggles to get what it wants or avoid what it so dislikes. For an infant exhibits will—some seem to be more determined or more bad-tempered than others—from the moment it is born. And this is uncontrolled. An infant is destitute of experience as yet.

At three months the muscles of its neck have grown strong enough to enable it to hold up its head. Its eye movements, too, are now co-ordinated, and it begins to look at things, learning to judge distance, partly by binocular vision, partly by experience. In short it begins to learn how to perceive. Further, instead of wanting to be left to sleep or to kick in its cot, it begins to take an interest in its own environment. It begins to wonder, again if its state of mind can be inferred from its behaviour, at the odd things people offer it with which to play, and which, like its own thumb, quickly find their way towards its mouth. Taste and tactile stimuli through the lips are the tests which an infant applies to any new object.

At the age of six months its muscles are sufficiently strong to enable it to crawl. Soon it can travel at speed across the floor. No complex balancing and no new reflexes are necessary for this, and now it is exploring the room, finding out what the things it sees are really like. Before long it is pulling itself up by its arms, and by the end of the first year its motor tracts come into action, and an infant can stand supported by the sides of its playpen or a chair. Walking, on the other hand, demands balance, and this depends on the rapid processing of information in its brain stem

66

and the integrated action of its cerebellum and sensory pathways in its cord. This needs time and practice to acquire. But the necessary machinery gradually comes into action, and by the end of the second year most infants walk unaided. Meanwhile control of visceral function has slowly been acquired.

When two or three years old, it begins to talk by operating the computer machinery which it has inherited and the speech centre genetic in its left frontal cortex. This results from unconscious imitation. It does not sit down to learn grammar, or strings of irregular verbs, like an adult struggling with a foreign language. Rather, it just listens and experiments, a first child usually late in learning to talk because it has no brothers or sisters to copy. For this reason, too, an infant born deaf never learns to talk, although it learns to associate lip movements of a certain kind with the meaning of the spoken word, and so learns to understand speech up to a point. But, not being able to hear anything, unable to hear even its own voice, it never talks without being taught, and never learns to talk normally. But the earlier a child starts to talk, the further it seems to get, other things being equal, in intellectual development, accounting perhaps for the fact that a second child and the later children of a family often seem to get further than the first. Talking is a stimulus to thinking, and thinking time lost in early infancy is not easily made up.

A new channel of communication has now opened up between an infant and its parent. It can now ask questions in an attempt to find things out. At first these mainly take the form of *What is so and so?*, questions often difficult to answer. Later come more awkward questions still, those of the *Why is so and so?* kind, questions still more difficult to answer in terms which its mind can understand. Indeed, odd ideas get stuck in an infant's mind very easily, and are responsible for many of the reactions and prejudices of later life, however much care and trouble is taken in answering its questions. In the first place, it cannot understand the most elementary relationship between cause and effect; so little has come within the ambit of its experience as yet. In the second, its mind at this stage works in terms of fantasy, in terms of things imagined, in much the same way as a primitive tribe reacts to things it does not understand. Shutting up a questioning child, because it is a nuisance, may have an unfortunate effect on the development of personallity. But an infant whose questions are answered to the best of adult ability, particularly if it is given plenty of material on which to exercise its imagination, suitable toys with which to play, and a few good myths to get on with, grows up free of fears and prejudices deep in its subconscious.

As age advances and experience widens, an infant begins to assert itself more and more. It now tries to mould its environment to its taste, and flies into a rage if frustrated in anything it wants to do, or get, or have, by circumstances or by other children; or retreats disgruntled when commanded repeatedly not to do something by its parents. Some discipline has been necessary from the start. No infant is ever allowed to do exactly what it likes—a mother's life would be unbearable if it was—but as a child gets older, there are more and more things that it wants to do, and correspondingly more things that it is not allowed to do; more and more things that are prohibited and more sanctions that are of necessity applied. Too little discipline breeds the spoilt child, the child lacking in self-control, its instincts and impulses running riot leading to lack of sense of responsibility and, paradoxically, to loss of freedom. It grows up a slave to its instincts and the victim of its own desires. Too much discipline, unthinkingly and rigidly applied, on the other hand, does harm. For self-will is the stuff out of which determination and personality are made.

Before long, instead of merely struggling to get its own way and expressing its own moods, a child becomes increasingly aware of those of others, and as it becomes aware of them, tends to take them on. If mother is frightened, her child is frightened too. If father is excited, his little boy gets excited. Just as in the past the infant has been physically dependent on its parents, and particularly on its mother, now it becomes emotionally dependent on both of them, imitating them and picking up what they say, trying to copy what they do, admiring what they like. (Hence the development of traits in a child which might otherwise have been thought inherited.) So, when worthwhile parents are lacking, mental development runs the risk of taking some unfortunate turn. A child may identify with the wrong parent, with a worthless renegade father, for example, or with a foolish self-indulgent mother; or, when parents are non-existent or remote, with some outstanding public figure or some character on the television screen. Love, more than anything else, is most likely to supply the material for the right kind of identification. But there is safety in numbers, and the more worthwhile people a child sees and gets to know, the better, other things being equal, it develops.

In the last act of the embryology of personality, an infant ceases to identify itself consciously with the person or persons whom it has been imitating, and takes over his or her or their characteristics as its own ideal of what it ought to be itself. In consequence it now becomes a mix-up within of what it feels it is, on the one hand, and what it would like or feels it ought to be, on the other, striving within itself after its ideal, however indifferent this self-imposed ideal may be. Hence the importance of a happy home in infancy and early childhood.

Childhood

The foundations of personality are laid during the three years that follow birth. Childhood builds on these foundations, and just as there is no absolute line of demarcation between the embryo and the foetus, so there is no absolute line of demarcation between the infant and the child.

Most people remember events in their lives such as birthdays and other great occasions, and sometimes trivial things that must have made a great impression at the time, and which can be confirmed as true memories, from round about the age of three. The still unfathomed mechanism of memory has been coming into action, recording accurately but intermittently as yet. Certainly most men and women remember themselves at the age of four or thereabouts, and remember themselves, too, as definite personalities with ideas and ideals of their own. Their parents, looking back, see them as miniature people, taking in some ways after them perhaps, because suggestion, imitation, and example had played such an important part in their development. Now, however, the child begins to know what it wants, and sets out to develop the necessary control to get it. Motives from within rather than from without now largely dominate its behaviour. It asks questions more and more. Every boy wants to know how a thing works; every girl how so and so is made. It begins to show off, too, as a way to establish its self-confidence, dominated by the ambition to appear grown up. Thus it gains sense of power, and this leads to rivalry and quarrels with other children. But the margin between fact and fantasy remains small. Children at this age often believe things they imagine to have happened, and readily escape into unreality. An imaginary friend is by no means uncommon.

At the age of four many are sent to kindergarten where they are taught to read and write. Others begin, or have already begun to learn at home. For, although all children learn to talk by imitating other people, they all need to be actively taught, first to read the written word, then to write the spoken one, and finally to write down in words the ideas which come into their heads. The rate at which they learn varies much, depending in part on the natural aptitude which they possess and in part on the skill with which they are taught. Those that learn to read and write early seem to get, from the educational point of view at least, furthest in the end. For reading is not only a source of knowledge—books open up a new world for a child and many get absorbed in them—but writing is a stimulus to thinking. And, as already pointed out, time lost at this age in respect of development of intellect cannot be made up later. Here we are on uncertain ground however. Pushing the development of intellect too hard may crowd out other aspects of personality development.

At the age of five the rat-race of compulsory education begins, and infancy, the period of dependence on parents and home, now give place to dependence on teachers and school. Further, a child now starts to make friends with other children, and these may come to mean more to it than its parents do or ever did.

Education should develop the potentialities of a child, physical and mental, as a member of the society to which it belongs, and in this extended sense is something far more than teaching for some occupation or profession. It includes character training and inculcation of moral sense, and demands the kind of handling that leads to a right sense of values which a purely intellectual training cannot accomplish. In practice this ideal is rarely achieved. In the first place, there is the increasing demand in a competitive world for factual and technical knowledge, and the consequent pressure of a complicated examination system, the hurdles of which must be got over by specified ages. This tends to crowd much else out, and those who cannot get over the hurdles lose interest until old enough to escape from school. In the second, there is the time factor. Many children have to travel long distances, and so most school hours are devoted to school work; there is little time left for games and other interests so important in character development. (Boarding schools in this respect, although they take children away from home, provide greater opportunity.) Thirdly, as there is no general agreement on religious matters—a decline in faith of all kinds is the order of the day—religious instruction in schools has been watered down to a minimum. The inculcation of moral values, which used to be anchored to religion, is in consequence now largely left out, although it is at this age that the foundations of individual conscience, on which society sets such store, are or could be laid.

Sexuality, like all other functions, develops well in advance of requirement, and even in infancy genital stimulation is a source of pleasure. As experience widens, this tends to get crowded out by other and extraneous interests. But it returns later, particularly in boys, in whom masturbation is normal, its ill-consequences psychological, rather than physical, and due to the odd ideas and repressed emotion associated with or engendered by it. In these days all reticence has departed, and every child is soon puzzled by what it reads and hears. Some are wisely helped. But instruction is difficult. Parents are embarrassed and shrink from it, while schools tend to leave it to them. Many children are still left to find out for themselves. But the way in which a child does become enlightened may have a profound effect on its attitude to sex throughout its life. This can colour its reactions, and determine its inhibitions, and in this way leave its mark on personality.

Adolescence

Round about the beginning of the teens the pituitary starts to secrete the gonadotropic hormones (p. 36). In a boy, secretion of F.S.H. leads to continuous spermatogenesis and seminal emissions; in a girl, to monthly ovulation. In both sexes, F.L.S. leads the gonads to secrete the sex hormones. These lead to the changes in the body whereby a boy is gradually transformed into and maintained a man, and a girl transformed into and maintained a woman. The alternation of secretion of F.S.H. and F.L.H. in the pituitary of a girl maintains the sexual cycle.

In boys the secretion of testosterone plays an important part in personality development, conditioning their reactions to experience in new directions. They become more self-confident and aggressive in their behaviour than they would have become for other reasons alone. (Inadequate secretion is associated with feeling of inferiority and general nervousness, and can even lead to stuttering.) The sexual instinct is, of course, inborn and, as we have seen, is present from infancy. Testosterone is, however, responsible for the sex drive that develops round about this age, although an exact relationship between desire and its secretion cannot be established. The latter seems to determine the general level at which sexuality is set. Psychological and other factors determine its fluctuations.

In girls the secretion of oestrogen also condition the reactions of the mind to experience in new directions, and every woman knows that her moods tend to vary with the phases of her sexual cycle. But it is much more difficult to assess the relative importance of physical and psychological factors in their psychosexual development. In general, psychological factors seem more and endocrine factors less important than in boys. Women are more complicated both physically and emotionally than men. This is hardly surprising. Every month a woman is on the brink of creation, and then all the complicated preparations for preganancy suddenly collapse.

At puberty both boys and girls both tend to shoot up suddenly in height. For oestrogen and testosterone both stimulate the growth of bone, although eventually they lead to the heads of the long bones fusing with their shafts, rendering further gain in height impossible. A child in whom the endocrine changes of puberty start early is above average height as an adolescent, but soon stops growing and finishes a short adult. A late developer in respect of puberty, on the other hand, is shorter than normal in his early teens but continues growing long after his contemporaries have stopped, finishing a tall adult. Further, as most inches are added to stature by growth of the long bones, the late developer has unusually long arms and legs. Sexual precocity, on the other hand, makes for short limbs. So at either end of the scale parents may have difficulty in finding clothes to fit a child who may be sorely embarrassed in consequence. Further, the protein building capacity of male hormone is much greater than that of oestrogen, and boys ten to develop stronger, bulkier muscles, and to possess heavier bones than girls. But they also vary much among themselves. While, for some as yet obscure reason, one boy is muscular and can lift weights and throw hammers, another is lightly built but can run long distances and is capable of infinite endurance.

The average age of puberty has fallen from sixteen or so to near the thirteenth birthday since the last century. The cause of this is by no means clear. Better nutrition has had something to do with it, and nutrition seems to play a part in determining the age of onset of it. Malnutrition delays it, as does disease of any kind. An over-fed child and a large child both tend to early puberty. But premature puberty, with the changes in appearance associated with it and its emotional reorientation, is three times more common in girls. For this reason a girl is often unfairly blamed for being precocious. Delayed puberty, on the other hand, is more common in boys, and a boy who develops late in this way may be troubled by fears of lack of manliness, and his difference from his contemporaries may lead him to lose confidence in himself completely.

Sexuality is homosexual in the first instance, and the free companionship up to this age between the sexes now gives way to antagonism. Boys begin to despise girls, and tend to gang together into groups, often aggressive and exhibitionist, under some chosen or self-emergent leader. Girls go off on their own. This phase is brief. Before long, and round about the school-leaving age, which at present stands at fifteen, homosexual gives way to heterosexual interest. A boy likes to show off to, and girls go out of their way to attract, the other sex.

Sometimes psycho-sexual development is arrested at the homosexual stage. But this has nothing to do, as might have been thought, with endocrine secretion as at present understood. Testosterone provides the sexual drive, but does not influence its direction. Male homosexuals have a normal endocrine constitution, and the administration of testosterone merely increases their homosexual desire. Genetic factors may have something to do with it. If one identical twin develops homosexual, the other, it is said, usually does so too. But, of course, they are likely to have been brought up under similar circumstances, and environmental factors and individual experience are more often blamed for homosexuality, particularly old-fashioned boarding schools and certain occupations and professions. On the whole it seems probable that homosexuality, like other aspects of psychosomatic development, is due to interaction between genetic predisposition, on the one hand, and individual experience, on the other.

The early teenage group today are faced with greater problems than their parents at the same age, and certainly with greater problems than those with which their parents' parents had to contend in their generation. Adolescence did not start then until their physical development was further advanced, they had left school, or anyhow their school days were nearly over, and the main hurdle of examinations had been side-stepped or surmounted. Today, with puberty standing at round about thirteen, these trials and tribulations all come together. The early teenager is faced with rapid growth, puberty changes, emotional adaptation to the facts of life, dawning interest in the other sex, and often as not some awful examination hurdle to get over, all at the same time.

Further, the gap between puberty and the freedom and responsibilities of adult life has widened. The middle teenage group are more grown up both physically and mentally than they used to be, the latter enhanced by better education. The average sixth-former and university student today are far more knowledgeable and sophisticated than before. Their fathers and grandfathers have made a hash of it: two world wars, and another war on still. They see poverty and starvation, social inequality and racial prejudice everywhere; hypocrisy in relation to sex in adult society, religious bunk abounding. They could and would fashion a new and better order. But they are still minors, possessed of knowledge without the opportunity to use it. Hence in part the feeling of frustration in teenage society, and its ills—promiscuity, drugs, psychopathic behaviour, revolt against authority, the demand for power. Their elders recognize these facts. A boy or girl, it is now generally conceded, is as much grown up at eighteen as he or she used to be at the statutory twenty-one. What they, the teenagers, do not realize, and cannot realize, is their lack of experience of things in general and of human nature in particular. There are short cuts to knowledge. But there is no short cut to that.

* * *

What am I? What ought I to be? We have now seen the answer which modern science gives to the first question, or rather the *description*, which it appears to give in reply to it, of the individual man and his nature, and the origin of both him and it, in terms of fundamentals and the way in which nature seems to work. But although science enables us to influence body-mind profoundly, and in future will certainly enable us to influence it still further—it has put new power into our hands—it does not tell us what man is in terms that the mind of man can understand, i.e. in terms of concepts which his mind can form. Still less does it tell us what he *ought to be*. The answer which the individual gives to that depends on the attitude to life which he has come to adopt as the result of living, and, if he is familiar with the findings of science in relation to it, on the interpretation he puts on them in the light of other aspects of human experience.

CHAPTER V

ATTITUDE TO LIFE

Religion—Science—Common sense—Philosophy—Morality
—Faith.

Man for some reason, although set up on animal pattern in body, is constituted differently in mind. While an animal lives in the present, except that every now and again it may start to hoard food or set out on migration, man lives in the future. In spite of being told to 'consider the lilies of the field which neither toil nor spin', he is always taking thought for the morrow, living emotionally in the future, either in short-lived confidence, in vague hope, or in anxiety or fear, but rarely in resignation to what he knows is really likely to happen. For he soon becomes aware of the disasters which may overtake him, and, as he grows up, more and more conscious of his own mortality.

Religion

To the sceptic all religious interpretations of human experience is little more than wishful thinking, born in primitive society of superstition and the necessity to propitiate an imaginary deity, and in more sophisticated societies by the need for solace, comfort and hope on the part of those not tough enough to face up to the changes and chances of life unaided. For security, it seems, is yet another basic human need, like food and sex and affection; and just as an orphan child longs for the love of parents who could guarantee its security, so man longs for the love of a God who could guarantee a happy ending to his life in spite of all the possible disasters which the world holds in store, the form of this guarantee, for the man who finds God, depending on the religion into which he was born or on the one to which he has been attracted by the same process of wishful thinking in

76

the course of growing up. 'Religion', said Karl Marx, 'is the imaginary realization of human perfection, the opiate of the people.'

Religion, too, has evolved, the sceptic would say, because it is a social as well as an individual necessity. According to Marx it was a device invented by the ruling class to keep the workers under, and it certainly provides intelligible sanctions for the control of instinct in human societies. The customs of a country are largely founded on its religion, or anyhow derived from a faith at one time generally accepted. For a national religion, with the idea of right behaviour anchored to it, promotes standards to which everybody is expected to conform, facilitates the maintenance of law and order, and makes for economy and efficiency. On this view religion is utilitarian only, utilitarian at a high price, however. It has been responsible for many of the wars of history, while until freedom of conscience was conceded as a human right, religious fanaticism was responsible for much individual persecution. On the other side of the balance sheet, religion, particularly evangelicism, was largely responsible for the social reforms of the nineteenth century. It abolished the slave trade, liberated the slaves, exposed child labour, reformed the factories, and rescued the abandoned children.

This is one view but, in spite of modern science which endeavours to explain man away as a super and rather peculiar animal, it is possible to take, as many people do, an entirely different view of the nature of man and his place in nature. For it can be held that a man's basic longing for security, although admittedly like food and the longing for sex and affection, an instinctive need, can become a longing for God. This longing, these maintain, is characteristic of the human race. There is in fact in this view a fundamental difference between man and the animals in that man possesses an inborn capacity to get to know God which is explained in Christian theology by the concept of man made in the image of God, fallen from perfection, and unable to struggle back to it unaided. Hence the Christian doctrine of the Redemption. Further, this inborn capacity to get to know God, like all other inborn or genetic capacities, varies in intensity in different people, and can be developed in them to different degrees during individual life. Hence the concept of spiritual vision into the transcendental, and the origin of the religious leaders of the world.

Between militant agnosticism, on the one hand—Victorian materialism is out-moded today—and convinced belief in some religion or another, on the other, there stands a vast body of uncommitted opinion, men and women unhappy about and unable to subscribe to organized religion, but far from agnostic or committed to a completely material outlook on human life. Further, as religion is in part man-made, being the interpretation which man puts upon his experience of living in transcendental terms and symbolic language, there have been, still are, and always must be, many religions, depending on the spiritual vision of their founders and the environment in which they lived, each with its own geographical distribution and particular symbolic language in which it speaks. But they all have something in common, and have arrived by different routes at much the same conclusions relating both to what a man is and what he ought to be.

Accident of birth usually determines the religion in which a man is brought up, and in general it is probably true to say that the local religion serves a man best in his relationship to God. 'Sir, we ought not,' said Dr. Johnson, 'without very strong convictions indeed, to desert the religion in which we have been educated.' But many are never educated in religion of any kind. Some of these, as life flows on, take to it. Others remain indifferent or actively sceptical. Further, within the same culture one man sticks to the religion of his fathers, while another abandons it or is converted to some other. In part this must depend on the way in which a man is made as the result of interaction between genetic and environmental factors. But many religious people say that their faith depends, not so much on reason or on their education, as on personal religious experience.

As knowledge widens, religion changes and adapts itself to increase in human experience. Theology claims to be progressive, like any other science. It has changed before, and will change again, and today the problem with which Christian philosophers appear to be confronted is that of linking up the basic need for God genetic in man, as revealed by clinical psychology, with belief in the existence of an objective God over and above man, derived from human reason, and God revealed, 'the word made flesh', based on traditional theology. They must also reconcile all three with the discoveries of the twentieth century.

Science

For science has painted an entirely novel picture of the universe which would appear to compel an entirely new concept of man's place in it as compared with that held little more than a hundred years ago. It is a concept with which the great religions of the world must come to terms, as the ambit of education widens, if they are to continue to cut ice. Just as the Gentile world had to adapt itself to the revolutionary teaching of Christianity, so Christianity and other religions today must now adapt to the revolutionary teaching of modern science.

The earth is no longer the centre of the universe. Rather, it is a small planet revolving round an unimportant star among millions of others on the edge of the Milky Way. Further, man no longer occupies a privileged position in nature. He has evolved, like every other form of life, at least so science says, and owes his dominant position in it to the natural selection of a succession of fortuitous mutations; and, as there are millions of other stars, and most possess planets, it is improbable that ours on earth is the only form of life existing. Indeed, it is improbable that man, as we know him, is the only form of 'man' extant. Further, although it is impossible to conceive of an absolute beginning or an ultimate end, the evolutionary idea, as opposed to that of creation, has invaded every branch of natural philosophy. Physics now describes the origin of the elements; astronomy, the birth of stars and the origin of the solar system; geology, the age of the earth; while time in retrospect is infinitely longer, and extension in both directions (i.e. into the atom and the cell and out into space) is infinitely greater, than was believed a few short years ago.

Modern science would also appear to compel the view that the individual is determined in all his main characteristics by an endless succession of combinations and permutations of minor cause and effect. These, operating according to the observed consistencies in nature (called by man its 'laws') are too complex to permit of prediction, and are written off as a chance. Chance in this sense would appear to have determined the meeting of his

parents, and also which of their gametes happened to fuse to engender the plan for his psychosomatic development laid at his
conception. Chance in this sense, too, and operating in this way,
not only determined his sex, his blood group, and the colour of
his eyes, but also that which both in body and in mind he could
eventually become. And chance also determined the environment in which the plan for him took shape, and thereby influenced its execution. For chance in the above sense determined his mother's health when pregnant, and the physical
environment into which he happened to be born. It also determined the psychological background of his childhood, now
admitted fundamental in the making of a man.

Further, modern science has also even tended to argue freedom of the will away. For, in view of the fact that all events in
mind are probably associated with physical events in the brain,
and as every physical event has an antecedent physical event, all
mental events must have antecedent physical events. So, at
least, the argument ran, and a man on this view no more orders
his own actions than a machine or a computer orders its. Rather,
they are all ordered for him by a relentless sequence of physico-
chemical cause and effect. On this view, determinism, freedom
of the will is an illusion. But this argument is now far from convincing in view of the fact that, according to modern science, a
principle of uncertainty with a consequent element of unpre-
dictability seems built into nature (p. 32). This concept leaves
room for free will, although it does not provide evidence for it.

Nor can science yet find evidence for purpose or design in the
universe, or any evidence of consciousness or mind outside the
higher animals and man. Nor can it find any objective evidence
for personal survival after death or any convincing evidence for
the intervention of a God in the affairs of men.

Common sense

On the other hand, although the teaching of modern science runs
counter to many religious ideas, it also runs counter to a very
large extent to that collective opinion on things in general which
is regarded as good, sound common sense.

The average man still lives pretty well convinced of his dual
nature, body *and* mind, rather than body *hyphen* mind, although

tied to his body, like a man on a horse unable for some reason to dismount. He does not really believe that he can be entirely explained away in terms of his genetic origin, environment and experience alone; that he is a different man today to what he was yesterday, as the result of just that little bit more of everyday experience. Rather, something permanent in him seems to carry on, and in spite of the evolutionary concept he feels fundamentally different to the animals. He may even still adhere to the idea of something immaterial which entered his body at some point in time, or gradually develops in it during his life; something in him aware, the machinery of his body permitting, of an absolute law over and above him and capable of choice; something capable of being made or marred during his passage through life, and capable perhaps in some way of surviving the death of his body on which his mind is based.

Further, although he may be doubtful about possessing a soul, every man still lives convinced that he is free, within limits, to control, or at least endeavour to control, his thoughts and actions. 'All the evidence is against it, Sir (free will)', said Dr. Johnson, 'all human experience for it.' And that, after two centuries of science and philosophy, is still the conviction of the ordinary man, the unrepentant verdict of humanity. No one in fact, although he may argue against it, seriously thinks that he has not got free will. He could hardly live a rational life if he doubted it, and it is a basic assumption of law. Free will must be accepted pragmatically and empirically as fact.

The concept of purpose in nature also dies hard in the human mind. Indeed, its antithesis, everything being merely due to chance, is somehow repellent to the human intellect. Man designed machines to serve his own purposes, and now finds, to his surprise, that many of them, the internal combustion engine and the electronic computer, for example, work on much the same principles as those on which his own body works.* Therefore, is it not reasonable, indeed rational and logical, to suppose that his own body, and also those of living things in general, were also somehow, in some way, at some time, planned? In that event mind must have come before matter, or anyhow before life started, instead of merely following in its wake as science would

* Bats judge distance on the same principle as that underlying radar.

suppose. So, may there not be something in the idea of progressive creation; even an element of truth in the religious teaching in regard to it after all? Any succession of purely random happenings, too, leads to chaos, but nature which, according to science, has evolved as the result of a succession of chance events is clearly very far from that. Rather, it appears essentially orderly. There are 'orders' of animals and plants, and these tend to reproduce their kind more or less accurately. The elements are arranged in a natural order in the periodic table. Even the universe with its galaxies and different orders of stars is systematic.

From the point of view of common sense science also paints a picture of the real world which is utterly incomprehensible; collections of charged particles revolving at high speed round other oppositely charged particles, leading to electro-magnetic waves which in turn cause changes in other similar systems in the human retina, leading to an image in consciousness of that which a man is seeing. Indeed, something just seen is not there as it was seen unless there is still someone there to see it. To common sense this is absurd, a problem which has troubled philosophers and led some to invoke the universal mind:

> There was a young man who said, 'God
> Must think it exceedingly odd
> If he finds that the tree
> Continues to be
> When there's no one about in the Quad.'

> *Reply:*
> Dear Sir,
> Your astonishment's odd:
> I am always about in the Quad
> And that's why the tree
> Continues to be
> Since observed by
> *Yours Faithfully,*
> God.*

* The first verse was written by Ronald Knox but no one knows who wrote the reply.

Nor does science, although it enables us to do extraordinary things, really explain anything in the way that man would like. In the past, it is true, it often seemed as if it did. Again and again it did succeed in explaining something which was not understood in terms of something which everybody could understand, because a man could form concepts of it in terms of his own experience. Explanations of this kind were really satisfying; for instance, that of the sequence of night and day in terms of the rotation of the earth. Anyone could understand that. Everyone knows that if something 'gets in the way' he cannot see an object. Indeed, at one time hope was raised, and some actually came to believe, that one day science would explain all natural phenomena in terms satisfying to the human intellect. But in these days it is abundantly clear that it never will. For the further science advances, the closer it gets to the fundamental incomprehensible attributes of human experience, space, time and energy, and the consistencies in the behaviour of nature which we call its laws, and the more *descriptive* and less *explanatory* in the mind-satisfying sense does it then become. Further, no longer is it descriptive in terms of concepts which the mind can form, but descriptive in terms of mathematic, which the mind has invented, as the result of man's experience of shape and number, and which, although it tells him nothing about the universe, enables him to manipulate matter and predict events in it. This suggests some relation between the human mind and the universe of which it is a part. But it is doubtful whether the mathematician, although he can do these things, comprehends them any better than the ordinary man. Or, put another way, science explains natural phenomena in terms of the incomprehensible, and in mathematics which man has invented, rather than in terms of concepts which he can form as the result of his own experience.

Nor does science take any account of values which play a large part in the conduct of human life. It does not enable a man to form judgments in aesthetics. It does not help him in moral predicaments. It furnishes him with no guide as to human relationships. For science can only take account of those aspects of experience which can be observed, weighed and measured. Values lie outside its ambit, and man today finds himself in an increasingly difficult position. The rapid rise of science has vastly widened the range of his experience, and put unprecedented power into his hands, but it has not yet provided him with any explanation of the universe or of his own place in it. Nor has it given him any guide as to when and how he should use this power in ordinary life, in peace or war, or in medical practice.

If the present tempo of progress is maintained, and man survives the consequences of his own inventions, this power is likely to increase still further. No one, it is true, can say for certain in what direction the next break-through is likely to come, but some discovery in the realm of the nature, as opposed to that of the working, of the mind is not improbable. For the claim that the individual mind depends *entirely* on interaction between heredity and experience is far from substantiated, and other factors with which science, for lack of method, has not yet come to grips, may enter into the genesis of it. The mystery of consciousness remains. There is much that is odd about personality, and the dominance of one mind over another. Hypnotism, the extreme form of it, has been known for two hundred years, but many phenomena related to it remain difficult to explain on the conventional basis of suggestion. Nor can some of the findings of modern work on para-psychological phenomena be ignored. The evidence for extra-sensory perception, one mind communicating with another other than through the ordinary channels of communication between man and man, by some mechanism in fact with which science has not yet succeeded in coming to grips, now seems fairly convincing. Further, although it can hardly be claimed that the results obtained invalidate the law of inverse squares governing the decline in the intensity of radiation from a source with distance, telepathy has been recorded at considerable distances, suggesting extension of mind outside the body on which the individual manifestations of it are based. Universal or group mind in this sense, if it exists, would modify our concept of the genesis of human personality profoundly.

Philosophy

Philosophy holds the ring and arbitrates in men's minds between knowledge based on objective observation and knowledge derived from subjective experience. It operates in the no-man's land between matter and mind. One sub-division of it is concerned with the nature of the universe, of which the mind of man is a part, as revealed by observation; the other with the best way for a man to live in it in view of his ignorance of its nature. But these two aspects of philosophy cannot be kept separate and distinct. The nature of the universe would, if man knew it, dictate how man, who is part of it, should live in it.

This first aspect of philosophy, the metaphysical, is concerned with the fundamentals of human experience, namely, space, time, energy, matter and natural laws, as revelaed by the scientific method, in relation to consciousness and mind. But modern philosophers are critical of much of the speculative work of past generations, and question the meaningfulness of many of the questions which men still tend to ask. It is useless to ask the nature of space, time or energy. We can describe them in relation to each other in mathematical language, which the mind of man has invented. But we cannot conceive of answers to what they are in terms that the mind of man, as at present constituted, could understand.

Further, modern philosophy would write off as meaningless much speculation relating to the relationship between mind and matter. Any form of dualism, except as a method of description in the face of lack of knowledge, is inadmissible. If two things are entirely separate and distinct, as body and soul are conceived to be, how could one influence the other; and, conversely, if two things influence each other, how can they be entirely separate and distinct? If two separate universes exist, they can never be known by, or make contact with, each other. Everything of which man can be subjectively conscious, or discover to exist objectively, must be related in some way to everything else of which he is, or has been, or can become, subjectively conscious. On the other hand, materialism, which attempted to explain consciousness and mind in terms of physical events in the nervous system, is as meaningless as the classical attempts to explain matter in terms of mind. Rather, modern philosophy inclines, as already pointed out, in the direction of regarding matter and mind as related to each other in some way of which the mind of man cannot form concepts, and therefore cannot understand. When a man sees something, there is physical change in his brain. When he wills something, there is a physical change

85

in his brain. Indeed, there is every reason to suppose that mental events cannot exist without concomitant physical events, and modern philosophy would deem it in the realm of speculation to assign priority to either.

Some hold that values in art and morals are objective. They exist apart from the subjective concepts of them formed in the minds of men. This, as we have seen, is the common-sense view. Others maintain that they are subjective only, born and bred in individual minds, the opinion of one man, one culture, or one generation, on this view, being as of much value as that of any other. Nor are philosophers agreed on the origin of knowledge. Empiricists hold that it all comes to man primarily through the senses with which his body is endowed. Rationalists maintain that some of it at least comes from within. It is innate in man, or anyhow in some men, and is reached by reason, meditation, reflexion and abstract thinking, or depends on intuition, that is to say, some sense which is not yet definitely recognized. The first view anchors all knowledge to objective experience. The latter, recognizing consciousness as *the* mystery, and the subjective position in which man is placed, exalts inner experience and sense of values in art, literature and morals, and widens out into philosophies of life, religious and otherwise, and into mysticism, medieval, modern and oriental, of which empirical philosophers and scientists tend to remain sceptical.

Among the former is the reaction against modern science and the empirical approach to philosophical problems now known as existentialism. According to Christian existentialists, man first exists in the mind of God. According to secular thinking, conscious man just exists, and then proceeds to think and doubt and shape himself. 'Man simply is', writes Sartre, the chief modern exponent in the latter school. 'He is what he wills, and as he conceives himself after already existing—as he wills to be after his leap towards existence. Man is nothing else but that which he makes of himself. That is the first principle of existentialism.'* This philosophy, as thus stated, restores free will, and man to his unique place in nature. It also provides the basis for and approach to psychoanalytical interpretation of individual

* *Existentialism and Humanism*, translated by Philip Marvel, Methuen & Co., London.

personality (existential psychoanalysis) which runs counter to the determinism of Freudian theory. But in so doing it would seem to fly in the face of many of the conclusions to be drawn from modern science. On the other hand, it translates into philosophical language the reaction of the plain man against the scientific interpretation of all human experience which to him seems so unsatisfying. It accords, in fact, in many ways with common sense.

Morality

Morality, that is to say the right way of behaving in situations demanding choice, in short what a man *ought* to do, or what the government *ought* to do, in certain circumstances must be achored to something. The word *ought* implies it, and there are only three things to which right behaviour can or could be anchored: the law of God, the welfare of other people, the concept of personal integrity.

Traditionally it is anchored to a natural law of right and wrong emanating from God. General principles only are laid down, as in the ten commandments of the Jewish law, and the individual is left to interpret them for himself in relation to the situation in which he is placed according to his conscience: military service, for instance, if at heart a pacifist; or having to vote on the issue of capital punishment. On this basis, as the believer's religion must of necessity be held by him to be nearer the truth than any other, its moral teaching is of necessity held by him to be superior to that of any other. In the Christian view, for instance, polygamy is wrong in any circumstances, moral philosophers within the Churches being tied in their judgment by the natural law of God.

It can be anchored to the welfare of society. According to this way of thinking an act is moral or amoral, not on the basis of any abstract principle, but whether in intent it makes for or militates against it—Jeremy Bentham's 'greatest happiness for the greatest number'. This was the philosophy behind the social reforms of the nineteenth century which have culminated in the Welfare State of this century. On this view morality is relative. What is right for one man in one social system may be wrong for another man in another social system, secular moral philosophers being free to base their judgments entirely on logic.

It can be anchored to the concept of the value of personal integrity, But the individual cannot be separated from society. He is a unit of it, and this fact provides the key to a secular concept of morality. A man's moral duty is to maintain his personal integrity in the interests of society of which he is a member, and this, it can be argued, is in the end of his own long-term interest. According to this concept intent is moral, if it maintains personal integrity and thereby furthers the interest of society, or at any rate does not cut across it; amoral if it impairs his integrity or harms society. A man's moral duty is not merely to be true to himself, worldly advice which Polonius gave to Laertes—that alone collectively tends to anarchy—but to endeavour, within the limits set by genetic endowment and environment, to make himself something to which it is worth while being true in the interests of society. Failure in this respect predisposes to neurosis, leading to mal-adaptation (p. 95), failure to see the necessity for it, to psychopathic behaviour (p. 101). Both are as much diseases of society as malnutrition, tuberculosis, and cancer.

The interests of self and society, of course, often conflict. Further, it may be difficult for a man to see what is the right course of action in certain circumstances. But the same difficulty arises in Christian ethics, and in practice there is much less difference between Christian and secular moral philosophy than might have been supposed. The command that a man should love his neighbour has the same practical implications as the humanist concept of man's duty to the society of which he is a member. According to both he should be prepared to sacrifice his health, and if need be his life, in the interests of others. Further, there are no absolute standards of morality either in Christian or secular ethics. What is right for one individual in one situation, is wrong for another in the same situation, or for the same individual in a different situation. The real difference between them lies in the nature of the reward. In the former this is perfection of an immortal soul. In the latter it is happiness in this world, maximum emotional satisfaction at minimum emotional cost, obtained by all right-minded well-adapted people by maintaining personal integrity in relation to society. Morality of this kind can be justified on a pragmatic basis. It works. Many, however, feel that right and wrong are natural laws as much as those which appear to govern the physical universe. They, and other values appreciated by man, just exist, like space, time and gravitation.

Faith

Science which has widened our knowledge vastly, must of necessity be right in general terms for the simple reason that its applications work in practice. The forces of nature have been harnessed to man's needs. The atom has been split to serve his purpose. Machines now do much of his mental and physical work. Astronomical events can be predicted. The implications of it in relation to the interpretations which man puts on his experience can therefore hardly be ignored.

On the other hand, science, although it works so well, does not really explain anything in the kind of way in which man wants things explained (p. 83). So the question arises as to whether there is or can be any other way in which he can get what so many want, any way in short in which he can get really to *know*. Here faith, if a man has it, or can develop it, provides the answer—faith in a personal God whom he can *know*, and through whom he can sense the answers born of the idea of God genetic in man of which physical science can take no account, and which philosophy argues away because the mind of man cannot, it contends, conceive of God. Values, however, cannot be denied. They exist in men's minds, many maintain, just as much as things exist in their environment. Further, it is clear that man does not possess cerebral machinery to enable him to form the necessary concepts to understand the real nature of things. A mouse does not possess the machinery to form the necessary concepts to understand man. Nor has a child developed the machinery to form the necessary concepts to understand things in relation to which its parents can form concepts and therefore understand.

Some argue that man, or anyhow some men, possess the cerebral machinery to be able to begin to understand God. The brain has in the course of evolution, these would say, reached in man, or at least reached in certain men, the point at which the mind developed on it can appreciate the existence of, and to some extent explore, a transcendental world over and above man, dualism the only language in which he can describe it. Perception of this transcendental in fact only registers in human minds, and perhaps only in certain minds. In them alone does the machinery of the brain permit it. This, of course, is speculation, but it can at least be suggested as an alternative explanation to wishful thinking for the religious sense genetic in most men, and peculiarly developed in some men. Further, if spiritual vision in this sense exists, it would of necessity be sometimes crowded out, like any other form of intellectual activity, by preoccupation with mundane things. Just, too, as a man is bound to be colour blind, if he does not possess the retinal machinery for the perception of colour, so on the hypothesis that spiritual vision in this sense exists, a man is bound to remain spiritually blind, if he does not possess the cerebral machinery for it. Many do not possess the cerebral machinery to appreciate music or to understand mathematics, although first class in other intellectual respects. Similarly, it can be argued, that the machinery for spiritual vision may be lacking in a man, although his mind is first class in all other intellectual directions.

The ordinary man must choose which road to follow. Genetic and environmental factors play a large part in his choice. Some, particularly those whose minds have been conditioned by their education into a scientific approach to problems, and particularly if they lack an artistic sense, tend to grow up sceptical of a transcendental. All religion, private or public, self-made or adopted, Christian or pagan, seems destitute to them of any objective evidence to back it. Others, made or brought up differently, react differently, and take what seems to them the higher road. Certainly the artist and poet, concerned with ultimate values, have little use for science. Their attitude to it is in fact one of bored indifference. It provides no answers to the really important questions which the mind of man insists on asking. They are only to be found in a transcendental world of subjective human experience.

The crux of the problem is the nature of mind in relation to the evolutionary sequence. Science maintains that matter came first, builds up life out of matter, then mind out of life, and then personality out of the reaction between heredity and experience. Alternatively, neither the universe nor man are the products of blind chance. Rather, both were designed. Mind came first, and exists independently of man. According to this view, the religious view, the individual mind must be thought of, not only in terms of interaction between genetic and environmental factors, but *also* in terms of the operation of transcendental factors of which science and psychology can take no account as yet. This demands faith, the conviction that there is some meaning to the universe in general and in human life in particular, apart from any evidence that can be adduced to support it at the moment, faith which Kant defined as 'knowledge sufficient for action, but insufficient to satisfy the intellect'.

The need for religion is no argument for its validity. It may be a biological necessity, essential to racial and national survival, without actually being true. In this brave new world, political idealism may take the dominant place it once occupied in society. But on the whole this seems unlikely. Many who do not subscribe to one of the great religions of the world develop a philosophy of their own. For the mystery remains, and as science advances, the mystery grows more and more mysterious. 'Every wise man has a religion', said someone, 'But no wise man says what it is.'

* * *

Weary of myself, and sick of asking
What I am, and what I ought to be.

What answer does science give to Arnold's second question, *What ought I to be?* It gives no answer, of course, except in terms of fulfilment of the plan laid for body-mind at a man's conception in relation to his mental and physical development. For science takes no account of values. He either therefore drifts through life in respect of his interpretation of it, thinks something out for himself according to his own ability, accepts the authority of others based on their collective experience, or follows the lead, as many have done, of one man in particular.

CHAPTER VI

FUNCTIONAL DISORDERS

Constitutional weakness — Nervousness — Neurosis— Hysteria—Psychopathic behaviour—Emotional states—The psychoses.

Perfect health is an unobtainable ideal. Possibly the nearest that can be got to a definition would be to say that a man is healthy when he has developed in body and mind up to average standards, and is capable of adapting himself to any physical or mental stress which 'the changes and chances of this mortal life' are likely to impose upon him. A really healthy man is also well adapted to knowing that one day he is bound to die.

Constitutional weakness

Some men, as the result of interaction between genetic and environmental factors, grow up better equipped for life in body or mind than others. While one is better furnished to cope with one aspect of life, another is better furnished to cope with some other. Equality of opportunity for all is necessary in order to achieve optimum development. But biological fact cannot be stretched to justify the political claim that all men are potentially equal.

All-round efficiency is associated with average architecture of body. Some are over-tall, height depending on the interaction of many variables. Genetic factors have much to do with it. There are tall families and short families, the pituitary and the gonads both secreting factors which regulate the growth in length of bone. Diet, too, affects it. Average height in this country is above what it was a hundred years ago, and is increasing in all countries where social conditions are improving. Others are over-weight in relation to their height due to a combination of heavy bones and bulky muscles, or truly obese in the sense that their ratio of stored fat to muscle protein is above normal, throwing an extra burden on their hearts and lungs. Obesity, as thus defined, is due to excess intake of calories over those required for muscular work and maintenance of body temperature, most people, for pleasure, social reasons or merely out of habit, eating more than their physiology demands. But obesity is not always due to over-eating. Rather, some people seem so made that they gain weight more easily than others. Whether constitutional obesity is really linked to cheerfulness—'Laugh and grow fat' is a common saying—is difficult to establish. But excessive height or weight sometimes makes it hard for a person to adapt himself to normal social life. An over-tall woman can be embarrassed by her height; a small man by his diminutive size. One obese person accepts his handicap with traditional cheerfulness, while another struggles unhappily, and often unsuccessfully, to slim in order to reduce his unattractiveness.

Sluggish circulation often leads to cold hands and feet, and the efficiency of the mechanism for the regulation of temperature also varies. Some cannot stand the heat; others the cold. Some cannot adapt to an irregular life; to meals at odd intervals, to broken sleep, to alternating periods of day and night duty. Others suffer from repeated headaches, attacks of indigestion, and irregularity of gastro-intestinal function. Further, the relationship between mind and body varies. Some are so made that emotional states have little repercussion on their bodies. After losing their tempers they can sleep as if nothing had happened. Others are less fortunate. Their bodies are disturbed too easily and long by the hang-over of emotional experience.

Mental characteristics vary even more widely than physical. One man is hard-bitten, thick-skinned or whatever metaphor is adopted to describe him; another over-sensitive, much too easily upset. One man presents a hard exterior but is unexpectedly soft. Another seems soft but proves, when the test comes, tougher than had been expected. Some are so made that they seem incapable of taking much interest in anything or being roused out of themselves. They do not seem emotional enough. If they could be roused, they might get something done. Others are too easily excited, or too easily depressed. Their emotional reactions to experience are excessive, and often interfere with their judgment with the result that they make mistakes, and then suffer from them, and in themselves, in consequence. Some are extrovert, full of friendship. They do not ask too many questions or expect too much of life, and are correspondingly adaptable to any situation in which they find themselves. Others are introvert, tied up in themselves, taking little interest in people in general, and puzzled by life and its problems. These find it difficult to adapt themselves to it, and may be correspondingly unhappy.

Nervousness

Fear is a common cause of not feeling well. For this component of the instinct of self-preservation leads, through the autonomic system, to changes in the body which put it in the best possible state to react to the cause of it. In animals this usually means fighting or running away. Hence the rapid action of the heart of which a man is so often conscious, the catch in his breath as respiration is stepped up, the dry mouth with cessation of digestive function, the cold sweat in anticipation of the need to keep temperature down, his hair standing on end (for protection in animals), and the tremor and tensing up of all the muscles in anticipation of the fight. But in human life there is seldom anything from which to run away and, except in dangerous sports, nothing about which physical action can be taken. So these reactions merely aggravate the emotional turmoil in a man's mind and, as we have just seen, some are more easily upset by their emotional states than others.

Further, just as some people seem to be born more intelligent or physically stronger than others, so some seem to be born more nervous or imaginative, or anyhow grow up more nervous or imaginative, than others. Indeed, some people come to live in a state of unreasonable fear, afraid first of one thing, then of another, imagining all the things that might happen to them, to those they love, or to those on whom they are dependent. Sometimes, too, they are so afraid of getting ill, and worry about it so much, that they may really begin to think that they have cancer, coronary disease, appendicitis, or something else about which they have read or heard. And the mere fear of disease can actually lead to pain. This may seem surprising, but all pain is an event in consciousness, and the idea of cancer of the lung, or the fear of getting 'a coronary', is a common cause of persistent pain in the chest. These people border on the neurotic, a more serious defect in personality development.

Neurosis

A normal man adapts himself with reasonable success to the traumatic experiences, the uncertain pleasures, and the potential risks of human life, and also to its apparent futility. He makes the best of his circumstances, whatever these may be. Realizing that, being human, he can't live just as he would like and be happy, he faces up to his situation, and adopts reasonable compromises as a basis for his behaviour, not necessarily at a very high level, but at one sufficient to enable him to fit into society and make his contribution to it. He has a conscience largely determined by his early upbringing. He maintains a sensible balance between self-interest and obligation to others, between duty to himself and duty to his neighbour. His behaviour is more or less intelligible, both to himself and to his friends, and predictable both to himself and to those who know him. The structure of his personality is satisfactory. He is steady and dependable within his limitations.

Conflicts, the stuff out of which neurosis is made, are inevitable in the mind of every man, their intensity depending on the vitality of his nature, the circumstances of his life, and the standards he has set himself, that is to say, on his conscience. In general the less vital his nature and the more pedestrian his mind, the less will be his conflicts; the lower the standard he has set himself, the less his difficulties. But the more vital his nature and the higher his standards, the greater—other things being equal—will be his difficulties in adapting himself to the life which he must or feels he ought to lead.

Religion, by setting standards to which he is expected to conform, can for this reason render mental conflict more intense, and some religious people only solve their problems by withdrawing from the world or by devoting themselves exclusively to the service of others. But for most people religion, unless conflict between faith and doubt complicates the situation, is a help rather than a hindrance. The feeling of purpose and faith in life, as opposed to the now common feeling of the futility of it, which it engenders, helps men to rise superior to their nature, and the religious are often happier than other people. Further, Christianity preaches resignation, that is to say, adaptation to difficulties and disappointments. They are part of the scheme of things, and to be endured. So, on the whole, there is less mental ill-health among the religious, particularly among Roman Catholics, it has been said, who accept authority in matters relating to faith and morals, than there is, on the whole, among thinking unbelievers who attempt to decide these things on some utilitarian basis. Religion provides discipline for those who cannot discipline themselves.

Some escape from their fears and difficulties by taking it out of themselves in work or play. Many intense hard-working people, and people differ much in the amount of energy they possess, are in fact escaping from their fears and conflicts; and up to a point this is legitimate, being nothing less than exaggeration of that sublimation of instinct into channels profitable to self and society which is part of normal psychosomatic development. Indeed, excessive preoccupation with one task or interest only borders on the pathological if it leads to neglect of duty, as when a man becomes over-preoccupied with his work or hobby at the expense of the welfare of his wife and family; if it leads, as to some extent it always must, to lack of interest in other things, and therefore to failure of development or maintenance of a balanced personality; or if the object of the obsession is peculiar in itself and born of maladjustment, as in the case of strange 'isms' and the pursuit of lost causes. On the other hand, a man who cannot become enthusiastic about anything, or run any one thing really hard, one whose mind is too balanced, although he may be as reliable as a rock, runs the risk of being dull and colourless. Besides, he tends to get nothing finished. Obsession is always to some extent dangerous however. For, when the task is done, faith lost, or the hope shattered, a man or woman, unless some other emotional outlet can be found, runs the risk of a nervous breakdown.

Other people grow up less satisfactorily. Genetic factors have much to do with this, as they have with all aspects of psychosomatic development. But unhappy circumstances and faulty management in early childhood, when, as we have already

96

seen, the foundations of personality are laid, are held mainly responsible. At that age development is proceeding fast. It is easy for some aspect of it to get crowded out, or partially left behind. So a child, instead of facing up to the traumatic incidents of early life, to the things it cannot understand, and to the conflicts between what it wants to do and what it is not allowed to do, may, if mishandled, repress them, and the emotion associated with them, into its subconscious.

Further, this way of reacting, if it continues, becomes, like any repeated activity, a habit. Then mental conflicts of various kinds, instead of being solved in the open, and the best available or only possible compromise adopted, are repressed into the subconscious—in ordinary language, forgotten. But they are still there, deep down in the mind, and although the neurotic person does not know it, much of his behaviour, and most of his motivation and his conscience, are in point of fact being determined by them. The more fears, inhibitions and complexes there are in a man's mind, the less understandable his behaviour seems to himself, and the less rational it appears to other people.

Neurosis is failure of integration in personality development, and no dividing line can therefore be drawn between normal and neurotic ways of reacting in the continuum of human personality with its infinite gradations. All men and women are neurotic in this sense to some degree, and much depends on their circumstances as to whether any defect of this kind ever gives rise to symptoms or leads to serious incapacity. Any man may break down when compelled to face up to unparalleled stress. Some officers, for example, who by any standards would have been considered the toughest type, broke down under strain and responsibility in both world wars. Conversely there are many who might not have grown up neurotic, had their lives worked out more satisfactorily. Physical ill-health can be a precipitating factor too. Most people stand up to mental stress better when they are fit than when they are out of sorts, anaemic for instance, sickening for something, or physically exhausted. Organic disease sometimes 'presents' as a nervous breakdown. The emotional factors which precipitate it vary widely. One breaks down, for example, when he finds himself unemployed, and has nothing in particular to occupy his mind; another when suddenly faced with a rush of work which he knows he will never get done. But the form of a nervous breakdown depends on individual personality and the nature of previous experience.

One feels desperately tired for no apparent reason, and again and again consults his doctor on this account. But his is tiredness of mind rather than exhaustion of body due to any physical cause. His ration of mental energy, and no man has an unlimited amount of it, is being used up uselessly on account of the turmoil in his mind due to repression of his conflicts. But he can often rise to a situation demanding action. When the external stimulus is sufficiently strong to over-ride motivation of subconscious origin, he may forget his physical tiredness altogether.

In another repression of emotional conflict leads to symptoms of a physical kind. A man seeks medical advice complaining of indigestion or loss of appetite and weight. He has got the idea into his head that he must be suffering from organic disease. Then even long and patient reassurance will often fail to convince him to the contrary. But the explanation of his symptoms is clear. Any turmoil in the mind drives the autonomic (p. 37) into action, and indigestion, loss of appetite and weight, and dysmenorrhoea and other gynaecological symptons, are easily produced by that.

Some cannot concentrate on anything due to the turmoil in their minds and become agitated and restless in consequence. A man cannot cope with his work; a schoolmaster, for example, with his pupils, or a business man with his employees. A woman may not be able to cope with her husband or her family, and after sparring with her doctor for a while, trying to take refuge behind some minor physical symptom, breaks down in a flood of tears.

Others feel worried or unhappy rather than ill. They cannot adjust themselves to their circumstances or to the inevitable limitations and frustrations of their lives. They are depressed by the apparent futility of existence, or they have emotional or physical difficulties in adapting themselves to the urges of their nature, and to problems relating to sex, marriage, family planning, birth control, and the like. Anxiety is the usual cause of frigidity and impotence.

Registration of events of any magnitude in memory, particularly those arousing emotional reactions, is physiologically inevitable. It can neither be prevented nor undone. But the mind can develop in such a way that it can prevent their recall to consciousness. A soldier may repress the memory of some battle ordeal, and never recall it to consciousness, although it may continue to trouble him in his dreams. Sometimes too, when a situation drastically demands escape, a man can lose his memory altogether, and wander at large, having lost touch for the time being with his own identity completely. Dreams, too, can lead to strange behaviour when consciousness is turned off in sleep. The classical example in literature is, of course, Lady Macbeth, with the murder of Duncan on her mind, gliding across the stage 'washing' her blood-stained hands. Unreasonable fear of open or confined spaces is often due to a frightening experience in childhood which has been 'forgotten' altogether.

Forgetting in the same psychological sense, the wish not to remember, may also be responsible for strange behaviour even when awake. Repression of some act of which a man feels ashamed may, for example, be partially repressed in the sense that only the circumstances of it, and not the act itself, or the act itself, and not the circumstances of it, are remembered. In the former, under the stimulus of the emotional hang-over associated with it, the circumstances, but not the act, may keep returning to consciousness, compelling him to return again and again to a certain place, for instance, though he does not know why; in the latter, compelling him to keep performing some act, perhaps, the meaning of which he cannot understand either. Indeed, his behaviour may worry him so much that he begins to feel that he is going out of his mind, until with help he succeeds in recalling what happened at that time.

Hysteria

Most people when they want something, and know or see that in decency they cannot have or get it, make the best of it and adapt themselves to the situation in which they are placed. On active service a solider may wish that he was ill or could be classed unfit. Then he would be safely out of it. After an accident a man may wish that he had been hurt. Then he might have got compensation. A widow, when her daughter seems determined to leave home, may long to be an invalid. Then she would have to stay and look after her. These are natural wishes which a normal man or woman rejects out of hand. The wish remains, but the man or woman resigns himself or herself to the situation in which he or she is placed, and few deliberately pretend to be ill in order to get what they want. But a neurotic person may repress his wish, be it to escape from a situation or to get something, and at the same time adopt the symptoms of some disease, which he has seen in someone else, read of in a book, or heard about on the radio, and now happens to serve his purpose, *subconsciously* and without seeing any connection between them and his wish. Thus he escapes from the unpleasant situation, or salves his conscience, with self-respect maintained. Hysteria, as this ability to keep two ideas dissociated in the mind is called, often amounts to a person getting what he wants subconsciously.*

Reactions of this kind, *conversion* hysteria, because a wish has been converted into a symptom, were common in the nineteenth century, during the First World War (at the beginning of which it was erroneously attributed to shell-shock), and for some years after that. Fits, paralysis, aphonia and other major symptoms are now rarely met, presumably due to better education, but minor ones turned on to gain emotional satisfaction remain common. Just as a badly brought up child gets satisfaction by taking it out of its parents by bed-wetting or obstinate constipation, so a woman may gain it by taking it out of a husband who has ceased to love her by exaggerating her headaches. She may even start attacks of some kind to make him stay at home. Reactions of this kind also figure large in the relationship between adolescents and their parents who, brought up in a different climate of opinion, often fail to understand and sympathize with the views and ways of the younger generation. In Edwardian times, a grown-up daughter, unhappy at home, would lose her appetite and refuse to eat, losing weight dangerously, but gain emotional satisfaction out of the family fuss she had precipitated.

* The word derives from the days when this condition was not understood and, being more common among women, became related in the medical mind to the uterus. Unfortunately, too, it has acquired an erroneous connotation in the lay mind, where it suggests excitement and loss of control when, as a matter of fact, having got what he wants, the patient settles down to enjoy his ill-health, and often exhibits *la belle indifférence* to everything else.

Everyone wants to be happy, although often happy in their own peculiar way, and happiness depends on gaining emotional satisfaction. But life for most people, particularly for women tied to the suburban home or tenement flat, and without the same opportunity for emotional outlets as men, may get dull indeed. Their children grow up and leave home, their husbands lose interest in them, and the daily round of chores goes on interminably. Further, they get little credit for working hard, and yet, like most other people, want to make a good showing. So it is not surprising that many women, starved of the emotional satisfaction which everybody wants, should often exaggerate any symptoms of the ill-health from which they happen to suffer, but in spite of which they work. In this way they gain emotional satisfaction. They are now long-suffering martyrs, both in their own eyes and in those of other people.

Psychopathic behaviour

Some grow up lacking in sense of responsibility. They have no or little conscience. They lack any feeling of obligation to society, and are content to profit out of it, seeing no reason why they should give anything back, happy, even proud, to live parasitic on it. These, the psychopathic, constitute a menace to society, and when they break the law by violence, stealing or sexual offences come into conflict with the State. Further, incapable of gaining satisfaction out of personal integrity, out of work, out of service to others, out of games, out of hobbies, they find an easy way of escape, particularly when they run on the rocks, in the dream world engendered by drugs.

The psychopath is in fact an adolescent who, as he grows up, fails to adapt himself to the ordinary conventions and limitations of social existence, and fails to develop a right sense of values in relation to life. He does not suffer from repression of conflict and complain of symptoms. Rather the defect in the structure of his personality is one of character. But, while a normal man makes some effort to control and compensate for any character weakness, or at least endeavours to conceal it, a psychopath exploits it to his own advantage, getting as much out of life as possible, regardless of other people. And his will can be strong. Hence the aggressive type. While the lazy man wishes he were not lazy, the psychopath exploits his laziness. The moral man has a qualm of conscience if he indulges in dishonesty, The psychopath tries to make money by dubious methods, starts pilfering, then stealing in a bigger way, or deliberately goes slow, and tries to avoid being found out. He makes the most of illness, or may pretend to be ill to avoid any job he particularly dislikes. The sensual man endeavours to control himself up to a point, and has some regard for the consequences of his acts. The psychopath could hardly care less. Perversion is often a misfortune rather than a moral failing, and many perverts suffer in their struggle with their perverted nature. The psychopathic pervert exploits his perversion to gain satisfaction, just as he would exploit anything else for that purpose, and runs the risk of collision with the law.

Genetic factors play an important part in the pathogenesis of the psychopath (p. 110). Some psychopaths are mentally inadequate. These commit the minor crimes, petty larceny and theft. Others are by nature manic (see next section), and commit regardless acts in their excitement. Others are abnormally aggressive or potentially epileptic.* The latter tend to commit the more serious offences. But upbringing and training also have a lot to do with it, particularly lack of discipline and authority in early life, opportunity, bad company, too much money, not enough work. Early puberty may predispose to it.

No dividing line can be drawn between psychopathic and normal behaviour, any more than one can be drawn between normal and neurotic behaviour. Most people are psychopathic, just as they are neurotic, to some extent, in the sense that they may be tempted at times to gain emotional satisfaction or

---

* Attacks of sudden loss of consciousness with or without convulsions have been recognized since the dawn of history, and were attributed at one time to possession by evil spirits. Now we know that epileptic attacks (which can also be induced by electrical stimulation of the cortex and by the administration of certain drugs) may be symptomatic of organic disease or idiopathic, that is to say, inborn, a manifestation of the way in which the individual is made. Further, these idiopathic epileptics tend to exhibit impulsive and irresponsible behaviour. Then it was discovered that this condition is associated with characteristic changes in the electro-encephalogram; also that some impulsive irresponsible people exhibited these peculiarities of the electro-encephalogram without actually having fits. Hence the concept of the epileptic psychopath.

material advantage at the expense of their own integrity and of the welfare of society. There is also the same relativity about it. A woman who has become a prostitute in one environment might not have become one in another. A man convicted of organized crime might have proved himself a first-class soldier. The recent increase in the number of psychopaths is in fact more apparent than real. In the old days they were kept under by long hours of hard work for low wages, and their temperament is at utter variance with the philosophy of safety first and the concept of social security which lies behind the Welfare State. The psychopathic mind demands an exciting outlet for its unbridled nature, and respectable citizenship hardly provides that. Many of the bravest soldiers of both wars were probably psychopaths by peace-time standards.

Emotional states

Emotional states, as we have already seen (p. 52) are associated with changes in certain centres in the brain stem, and can be induced both by consciousness of events, with an emotional connotation, and also by physical changes in the brain on which the mind is based. An emotional state can in fact be psychogenic or somatogenic. It is also commonly due to a combination of both causes. A man is more readily excited by good news if he has been drinking, and more depressed by bad news when recovering from an attack of influenza.

Depression and excitement can both be psychogenic; the former due, for instance, to a love affair gone wrong, or to an accumulation of emotional misfortunes; the latter to the prospect of the return of someone loved, to some imminent success or an accumulation of achievements. Further, excitement is, or should be, normal in youth, with the future spreading out ahead; depression inevitable in advancing age, as the future contracts and the past lengthens out behind. Depression and excitement can also both be somatogenic. Some drugs lead to depression. Others counter it, or lead to excitement. Disturbances of gastro-intestinal function, and the post-influenzal state, both lead to depression. Cerebral syphilis is a cause of pathological excitement. While some have grown up emotionally stable and run on an even keel, others are easily upset, up one day, down the next, their friends never knowing in which mood they will find them. Alternation of this kind is often associated with physical instability.

Some seem peculiarly predisposed to attacks of extreme depression by virtue of their physical constitution. That this predisposition is mainly genetic, rather than environmental in origin as in the neuroses, is strongly suggested by the fact that they tend to conform to the same red-faced, short-necked, broad-chested, so-called pyknic type. Further, there is usually a history of mental instability in the family. Most too, tend to be extrovert, a mental characteristic which we associated with this physical type, the hail-fellow-well-met. Then suddenly, for no apparent psychological cause, a man of this kind is overtaken by depression, which is therefore said to be endogenous (i.e. coming from within rather than due to any cause acting from without). Indeed, it seems fairly certain that in these endogenous attacks the emotional centres in the brain stem are affected physically, as in bromide poisoning and post-influenzal states.

The mind is retarded. The man—they are usually men—cannot think, plan ahead, or cope with his problems. Life has lost its attraction, and hope dried up. Further, although he ought usually to know from previous experience that he is merely going through a dark tunnel, and will emerge one day at the other end, he cannot see it that way. For the moment he is living in a world of eternal misery of his own creation and, to use an old-fashioned word, is alienated altogether from his normal self.

Comparable attacks of unaccountable excitement, mania as it is called, also occur, although less commonly, in the same physical type. Sometimes, it is true, these seem to be precipitated by infection or by something exciting that has happened. Far more often these also start for no apparent reason. Again they are endogenous, and their pattern is always much the same. The man—again they are usually men—gets increasingly excited, and keeps dashing from one thing to another, starting everything, finishing nothing, his conversation a continuous stream of disconnected talk. He never wants to go to bed. Life has become too exciting to bother about sleep. He is tireless. Every moment must be lived, and the delusion that something grand has happened may come to dominate his mind and determine his behaviour. This may render him dangerous to himself or to other people.

In these conditions the patient is psychotic rather than neurotic, that is to say he is living in an unreal world. It may be feasible to give a neurotic some insight into his behaviour, and help him to adopt a more reasonable attitude to life; possible to help a person, whose depression is psychogenic, back to happiness. But it is useless to try to make a man in an endogenous depression see that the world is not as black and hopeless as his mind paints it; equally useless to try to convince another in a state of mania that the event about which he is so excited has no foundation in fact.

The opposite physical type, the asthenic, the lank and weedy with poor circulation and sometimes cold blue hands, introvert, shy, uncertain of themselves and solitary, are liable to psychotic breakdown of a different kind which tends to occur in rather earlier life. Again the predisposition seems genetic. Again there is often a history of mental instability in the family. If one identical twin develops schizophrenia, as this form of mental breakdown is called, the other often does so too. But environmental factors, particularly the way in which a child is brought up (another possible explanation of schizophrenia in twins) are important, and the mechanism of the development of the schizoid personality has been much studied. As in the neuroses its psychogenesis depends on dissociation. Again a bit of the mind has been split off. But, while in the neuroses this dissociated part disturbs consciousness, because it is not under the control of the will, in schizophrenia it has gained control of it. Whether schizoid predisposition actually leads to psychotic breakdown depends on interaction between genetic and environmental factors. One schizophrenic would not have broken down, had he not been exposed to stress. Another man would have done, if his life had been less sheltered.

The first symptom is usually withdrawal from the world in attacks of confusion and dejection with consequent depression. They must be left alone. Soon they begin to get suspicious. They are being watched. Before long they begin to suffer from delusions, often due to dissociation on two fronts, both from self and from society. The former leads to delusions of pre-existence or detachment from the body to which, in the course of development, the mind normally becomes anchored. The latter leads to withdrawal into a world of fantasy in which the real one ceases to matter, and in consequence of which the untreated schizophrenic loses affection for his friends, and may laugh at tragedy, although still understanding its meaning. Sometimes a particular delusion determines behaviour. Some believe they are being persecuted; others that they have made some great discovery, and live in agitation because the world refuses to accept it. Some set themselves impossible tasks which they can never finish, like Betsy Trotwood's Mr. Dick who could not keep King Charles out of his 'memorial'. Others wander about in strange clothes, imagining themselves someone other than they really are. Some withdraw into themselves and sit all day in dejection. Others stand in some grotesque position for hours without semblance of fatigue.

Insanity remains puzzling, and at times seems akin to genius. A high proportion of the Italian artists, Viennese musicians and German writers had bouts of insanity, and there is something strange about the dissociation of the schizophrenic from his physical self. Further, the mind cannot be explained entirely in terms of interaction between genetic predisposition and experience. To claim that is extravagant, and there may well be, as already pointed out, factors operating in the genesis of the normal mind with which neither physical science nor clinical psychology have yet come to grips; and, if factors at present unknown enter into the genesis of the normal mind, they are bound to enter into the genesis of the abnormal mind. Some claim that in schizophrenia, and under the influence of psychedelic drugs, the mind 'soars into worlds unknown'; that the schizophrenic possesses vision denied to normal men, a view reminiscent of *The World of the Blind* (H. G. Wells) in which the man who could see was certified insane. But there is no evidence that any psychotic experiences or any of the hallucinations engendered by drugs are anything more than extension of that exaggeration and distortion of human experience which occurs in the dreams and nightmares of normal people.

*　　　*　　　*

Physical constitution varies widely among men, and the particular kind of mental breakdown to which some are predisposed is determined during the early years of life when the genetic plan, whence a man is derived, is conditioning the development of his mind under the stimulus of experience. But there are no clear dividing lines between normal, nervous, neurotic and psychotic mental states. Rather, a person can move backwards and forwards from time to time between them, the manifestations of mind being a continuum on which man imposes his classifications in order to try to help him understand it. The neuroses and some cases of depression are mainly psychogenic. They are due to emotional trauma, the body playing little part in their pathogenesis, and although the symptoms associated with them are often of a physical nature, they are always of the kind which the mind can turn on by interfering with the working of the body. The psychoses, on the other hand, are largely somatogenic in the sense that some peculiarity of physical constitution, determined by the genetic plan laid at conception, so conditions psychosomatic development as to predispose that individual to breakdown in circumstances which would not disturb a normal man.

CHAPTER VII

ORGANIC DISEASE

Genetic defects—Malnutrition and deficiency disease—
Physical injury—Chemical poisoning—Infection—Allergy
—The not-yet-understood—New growth—Blood pressure—
Degeneration—The psychosomatic concept.

In theory it is impossible to maintain a rigid distinction between functional disorders and organic disease for the simple reason that plans laid at conception, and leading to normal development, merge imperceptibly into plans predisposing to abnormal development. But in practice this distinction can be, and, for practical purposes, is maintained. For while functional disorders, with the exception of psychotic states (which some would also classify as organic), are non-progressive and non-lethal, organic disease is often progressive, and sometimes lethal. Early diagnosis can be particularly important.

In the former, body-mind is 'going badly', different men like different cars being capable of different standards of performance, and not all human bodies, like man-made motor cars, are equally well driven. In the latter, the working of the body is radically at fault, there is structural change in the body in most cases, and it would be convenient if we could define organic disease in terms of that. But we cannot. For body-mind is a physico-chemical set-up, the working of which depends on transient change and the structure of which depends on its more permanent chemical arrangements. The former sometimes goes wrong without affecting the latter, as in diabetes, for instance. But organic disease is in point of fact usually associated with structural change. This can often be detected during life, and demonstrated in the body after death.

Genetic defects

Body-mind may get off to a bad start. One infant in every twenty

108

is born with some abnormality, and one in every seventy-five, it can be said, sufficiently abnormal in some respect to demand action of some kind sooner or later. Some of these congenital defects are genetic. We know that because they are inherited.

Some genetic defects are unimportant or only matter in certain circumstances. Colour blindness, due to a dominant gene, is usually only discovered when a man is tested for a job demanding colour vision. A few are advantageous in a sense. Achondroplasia, one variety of dwarfism, provides the short-legged, square-headed clown and, as it is due to a dominant gene, there are often several in one family. All are notoriously quick on the up-take, like Miss Moucher in Dickens's *David Copperfield*.

Other genetic defects are potentially dangerous. Familial polyposis of the rectum, due to a dominant gene, predisposes to cancer of the rectum; spherocytosis, a condition in which the red corpuscles are spherical, also due to a dominant gene, to their over-rapid destruction, and therefore to anaemia. In Huntingdon's chorea a gene which affects the development of the brain leads to uncontrollable movement of the limbs. It has been traced down twelve generations. Conditions due to a recessive gene only turn up occasionally; congenital deafness, for instance, which leads to mutism, because the child cannot hear and copy speech; and some odd disorders of the chemical working of the body, for example, porphyria which led to the madness of George III.

These conditions, dominant or recessive, can all be inherited through either parent, and occur in boys and girls in the same proportion. Others are transmitted through the female, but are only inherited by the male, the best example being afforded by haemophilia which runs through the royal families of Europe. The blood fails to clot as it should, creating the risk of serious haemorrhage. So haemophilics seldom live to marry, and were haemophilia not kept constant in our midst by new strains starting as quickly as the old ones are bred out, it would itself die out.

Genetic disease may also be due to chromosome abnormalities. Mongolism, a variety of mental deficiency associated with physical features resembling those of the Mongol race, is due to an extra chromosome, and other congenital defects may prove to be due to a similar cause. Further, in the formation of the germ cells, instead of one sex chromosome passing into each daughter cell, both may pass into the same one, leading to spermatozoa of genotype XY and O, and to ova of genotype XX and O. Odd things now happen when a gamete of one of these types meets a normal one. The fertilized ovum will either have an extra chromosome (i.e. 47 instead of 46) and be of genotype XXX or XXY; or be one short (i.e. contain only 45 instead of 46) and be of genotype XO or YO. The former leads to a male child, feminine in appearance and mentally retarded; the latter to a female with webbed neck, dwarfed stature, and malformation of the heart, who fails to mature and remains mentally retarded.

Sex in fact is not absolute. No clear dividing line can be drawn between the sexes, true intersex appearing to be due to abnormal sex chromosome content of the somatic cells, accounting for the masculine type of female and some 'female' athletes. Further, there seems to be a connection between psychopathic behaviour and sex genotype. Psychopathic males of genotype XYY and XXYY show significant differences in respect of the age of their first conviction, the type of crime committed, and the criminal records of their siblings, as compared with psychopaths of normal XY genotype. This suggests that their personality defect is linked with the two Y chromosomes, rather than the consequence of environmental factors in their upbringing, as might have been supposed.

No absolute dividing line can be drawn between genetic and acquired disease. Many people start life predisposed to succumb to one of the risks in the environment into which they are born, while the mortality of the male at all ages due to all causes is greater than that of the female. Further, in view of the fact that certain environmental factors, notably cosmic radiation, predispose to mutation, genetic disease itself can in a sense be acquired. But the distinction is practical, and the known risks to which man is exposed, although again no absolute dividing line can be drawn between them, can be divided into groups, most of which can, in certain circumstances, affect the unborn child leading to the acquired, as opposed to the genetic variety, of congenital disease.

Malnutrition and deficiency disease

An infant *in utero* is nourished through its mother's blood. A woman living in poor circumstances starves herself to feed her child but, if she is anaemic due to lack of iron in her diet, it too is born anaemic. Further, she keeps it supplied with oxygen through her blood, and during the delivery of a breech presentation, compression of the cord by the after-coming head may lead to serious and sometimes fatal failure of its oxygen supply before pulmonary respiration has had a chance to start.

A prisoner may go on a hunger strike in protest, as the suffragettes did just before the First World War and the Irish nationalists soon after it. The Mayor of Cork starved himself to death, and developed scurvy before he died. (No one has yet deprived himself of water.) Normally starvation is due to famine or to over-population in relation to food supply or to some combination of the two; or to the result of accident, such as shipwreck; or to war, as during the siege of Paris in 1870 and that of Kut-el-Amara in 1916.

For the human body must be maintained, an average adult in ordinary work requiring 3,000 calories, 70 grammes of protein, and three pints of water every day; also 200 c.c. of oxygen a minute at rest, and certain salts, minerals and vitamins. A child, on account of its large surface area in relation to its weight and volume, and consequently more rapid loss of heat, needs to maintain a higher metabolic rate. While a grown man in full work requires about thirty calories per kilogram of his body weight, a new-born infant demands nearly a hundred. For the same reason an infant loses water by evaporation quickly, and wants a relatively large quantity, particularly if it is losing it in any other way as well, as for instance, in vomiting and diarrhoea. An insufficient supply of food at any age leads to malnutrition and loss of weight; of water, to dehydration and loss of weight. Lack of vitamins leads to deficiency diseases; of Vitamin D, to rickets (common during the industrial revolution); of Vitamin C, to scurvy (at one time the rule on long voyages); of Vitamin A, to night blindness; of Vitamin B, to beri-beri, a form of paralysis associated with heart failure and oedema. Shortage of iron leads to anaemia and of calcium to rarefication of the bones.

Physical injury

The infant *in utero* is well protected, the only serious traumatic risk being that a loop of umbilical cord might become twisted round one of its limbs and obstruct its blood supply. Then its development lags behind that of the other. At birth mechanical compression may injure the skull and underlying cortex, particularly if forceps are applied to accelerate delivery. This is one of the causes of the spastic child.

Throughout life everyone is exposed to the risk of physical injury, particularly in certain occupations and in all dangerous sports. Some, too, lack foresight and are more prone to accidents than others. Further, the body does not always seem quite sufficiently strong in some respects, and may succumb to some internal strain; when a man prolapses an intervertebral disc, trying to lift a heavy weight, for example; or fractures a small bone in his wrist, playing a stroke out of a bunker; or ruptures his tendo Achilles, getting off his marks at the sprint. Far more often injury is the result of an accident. Externally applied force divides an artery or vein, ruptures capillaries, severs a nerve, fractures a bone, dislocates a joint, or perforates a hollow organ. Any severe accident also leads to fall of blood pressure and traumatic shock.

The injuries which the body may sustain are infinite in their variety. But its inborn reactions to them, tending to repair damage done and restore the *status quo*—reactions which have developed in the course of evolution—are consistent. Blood begins to clot, tending to stop haemorrhage by plugging the wound, while the fall of pressure associated with shock minimizes the bleeding; and lost blood is gradually made good by the marrow stepping up its normal rate of blood production. Any cut soon starts to heal (particularly if its edges are drawn, and if necessary stitched, together) by the formation of fibrous tissue leading to a scar, while a bone mends and, if kept in the right position, mends without deformity by forming new bone which unites the fragments. A divided nerve regenerates by the cut end slowly growing down the old route to reach the muscle which it has been its function to supply. But in a really serious injury, division of a main artery or perforation of the gut, for example, the body fails to cope unaided with the situation. Whether the injured man recovers depends on a balance between the nature and extent of his injuries, the reactions of his body to them, the amount of blood which has been lost, and whether help is available in time.

A man can keep his body temperature down to normal even when that in the shade rises well above it, as is often the case in tropical climates. This he does by sweating. The rapid evaporation of water, owing to the heat required to effect it, lowers temperature in its immediate vicinity. So, if for any reason a man in these circumstances stops sweating, his temperature starts to rise, and he dies of heat stroke at about 110° F.

Slight exposure to heat reddens the skin. More severe exposure raises blisters due to accumulation of fluid between dermis and epidermis. More severe exposure still destroys the dermis and underlying tissues, and burns of this so-called third degree lead to severe shock. Burns also lead to the absorption of toxic substances due to local destruction of tissue. This leads to a febrile reaction. The reactions of the body to burns are identical with those to physical injury but, as would be expected, are slower in coming into action. Local repair may take a very long time indeed.

Ionizing radiation, that is to say, radiation of sufficient energy content to knock electrons off atoms leaving them charged, also damages the human body. Ultra-violet light falls into this category, and moderate exposure to it reddens the skin, while excessive exposure raises blisters, like a burn of the second degree, and reflected from snow can cause serious damage to the retina. Ionizing radiation of other kinds is more dangerous still. Many of the pioneers of X-ray diagnosis developed anaemia, due to destruction of their bone marrow, and chronic burns, in which malignant change developed (p. 122), before these risks were realized, and the necessary precautions taken against them. Further, over-exposure to X-rays, to radio-active isotopes, or to radium, may lead, it is now known, to leukaemia (p. 122), to mutation (p. 30), and to sterility, to eunuchism in men and to a premature menopause in women. X-ray treatment is often followed by nausea and sickness with rise of temperature and general malaise.

Atomic explosions of any kind lead to sudden mass liberation of ionizing radiation, and as the result of those inflicted on Japan in 1945 many died of acute radiation sickness or of leukaemia at a later date. But the margin between exposure, leading to mutation, and exposure, leading to sterility, is small, and the genetic consequences of the bombs dropped on Nagasaki and Hiroshima do not appear to have been as great as was feared at first. The level of ionizing radiation in the atmosphere has, however, risen with successive atomic tests by the great powers, increasing the mutation risk. Further, all atomic explosions lead to radioactive fall-out, the most dangerous component of which is a radio-active isotope of barium, an element which the body treats as calcium. So it may be deposited in bone, predisposing to malignant disease.

Chemical poisoning

Substances with a deleterious effect on the body can be inhaled in the air we breathe, swallowed in the water we drink, ingested in the food we eat. Many substances used in medicine have unwanted effects, while dangerous chemicals are used in industry and agriculture. The latter, unless due precautions are taken, can find their way into the body through hands or lungs, and in the case of those used in agriculture or to preserve our food, through our intestinal tracts. They can also be taken with suicidal or used with criminal intent. Further, a number of chemical substances have long been taken for pleasure, and now, as the result of recent advances in organic chemistry, new ones of this kind are being rapidly discovered.

The air we breathe is contaminated by the smoke from coal furnaces and by the exhausts of internal combustion engines. The former contains sulphur dioxide which, like chlorine and phosgene used by the Germans in the First World War, is irritant to human lungs, leading to bronchitis and predisposing to pneumonia. The latter contains carbon monoxide which appropriates haemoglobin, leading in sufficient concentration to asphyxia—hence the danger of keeping the engine of a car running in a small garage—and also certain hydrocarbons which predispose to cancer of the lung, the incidence of which is greater in cities than in country districts. Further, by smoking a man contaminates still further the air he breathes, and, as everyone now knows, smoking also predisposes to cancer of the lung.

Other poisons act by interfering with the chemical machinery of the body. They undermine some vital link or jam its machinery somewhere, many being remarkably specific in their action. The most dramatic is hydrocyanic acid which the Nazi leaders concealed in their mouths, and used to commit suicide after the Nuremberg trials. For it interferes with the enzymes which effect oxidation in the body, leading to almost instantaneous death. Lead, which is much used in industry, and gets into drinking water fed through lead pipes, interferes with the conduction of the impulse in peripheral nerves and leads to paralysis. Some toys imported from abroad are painted with lead-containing paint, and are dangerous to children. Methyl alcohol affects the optic nerves, and may lead to blindness. Other substances, many of them used in industry, pick out motor or sensory tracts in the nervous system. Lead also affects the intestinal tract, and causes colic. Arsenic leads to chronic diarrhoea. This resembles natural disease so closely that it has been used with criminal intent.

All the potent drugs used in medicine are poisonous in overdose. General and local anaesthesia are controlled poisoning for therapeutic purposes. The barbiturates, which promote sleep and depress respiration, are often taken with suicidal intent. Digitalis stimulates the heart, but taken in over-dose leads to fibrillation of the ventricles and sudden death. Curare, which paralyses all motor nerve endings, is used to prevent convulsions in the treatment of tetanus and in electric 'convulsion' therapy (p. 176). Many drugs, too, although potentially safe in their therapeutic intent, have unwanted side effects which limit their use in practice. Cortisone, for instance, until recently often used to inhibit reactions to the antigen in allergic states—other immuno-suppressive drugs are now mainly employed—not only increases the risk of infection by inhibiting the reactions of the body to it, but also leads to retention of salt and water, and to consequent increase in body weight and, if pushed, to clinical oedema. Some of the antibiotics interfere with the formation of the blood, and some of the tranquillizers have a toxic action on the liver leading to jaundice. But this does not happen in all cases. Rather, it is a matter of idiosyncrasy, some people being so made that they are peculiarly susceptible to them.

Drugs taken for pleasure have a deleterious effect on body-mind. Alcohol releases inhibition, making a caricature of a man before in an acute alcoholic bout it leads to confusion and ulti-mately to coma. Persistent consumption over a long period, possibly by interfering with diet and causing chronic vitamin deficiency, leads to peripheral neuritis and fibrosis of the liver (cirrhosis). It also leads to progessive mental deterioration. Opium and its active principle, morphine, and a chemical derivative of the latter, heroin, all lead to detachment from reality and, if taken for long periods, to lack of motivation, slovenly habits, and progressive moral deterioration. To what extent *cannabis* (Indian hemp or hashish) and the new psyche-delic drugs such as L.S.D. and S.T.P., which engender hallu-cinations comparable to those experienced in schizophrenic states, are to be regarded as poisons, and the taker of them to be poisoned, is a matter of definition.

The reactions of the body to chemical poisoning are as con-stant and consistent as those to physical injury. Again, too, they are inborn. Many chemical substances are rejected by vomiting, while those which escape that, or have by-passed the protective reactions of the stomach, because they were injected, are ren-dered innocuous by the liver or excreted in the urine. Indeed, the body seems to 'know' how to deal, not only with many sub-stances it has never met before, but with many which it seemed most unlikely that it would ever meet. Further, it improves with practice. A morphine addict can tolerate a dose which would kill an ordinary man. The body can in fact defend itself against chemical poisoning due to accident or indiscretion, although again, as in physical injury, there is a limit to its capacity in this respect.

Infection

Infection can occur *in utero*. German measles during the early weeks of pregnancy may lead to foetal malformation. A syphilitic mother can infect her child.

The body is born 'sterile', although its orifices, its protective covering, and its colon, soon become infected, that of the colon leading to the synthesis of vitamin B., an example of symbiosis comparable to the digestion of cellulose in the gut of herbivorous animals. The small intestine and the lungs, although open to the air, remain sterile throughout life.

All other infection is pathological in the sense that it tends to alter the structure of the body or upset the way in which it works. Fungi and insects irritate the skin. Intestinal parasites compete in the gut for the food a man needs. Pathogenic spirochaetes and bacteria penetrate his mucous membranes, and either live and multiply in his blood, or bale out in a certain part of his body, competing generally or locally for the substances on which his body as a whole, or that particular part of it, depend. A few set free substances which have a deleterious effect elsewhere. Diphtheria bacilli, for instance, stay put in the throat, but liberate a toxin which has adverse action on the heart. Tetanus bacilli get into a wound, but get no further. From the security of that they liberate a toxin which reaches the nervous system and sensitizes it to stimulation, leading to generalized convulsions.

The body reacts to infection, just as it does to injury and poisoning, the particular reaction being largely determined by the nature of the invading organisms and their method of attack. To local infection it reacts by inflammation, i.e. engorgement of vessels, leading to heat, redness, swelling, pain, and concentration of white blood corpuscles in the neighbourhood; to general infection by rise of temperature with all its well-known symptoms, namely, sweating, shivering, headache, loss of appetite and general malaise. Infection of this kind is said to be acute, and fever is as important in overcoming general infection as inflammation is in overcoming local infection. Further, much is going on behind the scenes of which a man is completely unaware. For all pathogenic organisms, when they get inside the body, stimulate the production of antibodies which tend to destroy them, while diphtheria and tetanus toxin stimulate the production of antitoxin. This latter neutralizes toxin in the body much in the same way as alkali neutralizes acid in a test tube.

Local infection of an acute kind, usually due to staphylococci or streptococci, leads to the destruction of tissue and the formation of an abscess. This comes to a head and bursts, restoring the *status quo*. But the reactions of the body may fail to prevent

bacilli getting into the blood. Then, before the advent of chemotherapy, death from general septicaemia resulted.

When organisms slip in without stimulating any immediate
opposition, the body reacts less violently. Further, attack and
defence are now largely local, the latter taking the form of
fibrosis, as in the healing of a wound, cordoning off the invaders,
rather than congestion and leucocytosis, making for their destruction. And there is little systemic reaction. So infection of this
kind, instead of coming to a head and dying out, tends to wander
on and become chronic. In short, there is now cold war within
the body politic. Before the advent of chemotherapy, tuberculosis, for example, would persist in a lung, joint or kidney, for
years before coming to a head. Syphilis, due to a spirochaete
which chooses the heart, spinal cord or brain for its habitat,
although rarely a cause of death, can remain active in the body
throughout a man's life.

Other infective diseases are due, not to bacteria but to viruses;
in man, influenza, for example, and the common cold, measles
and mumps, shingles, small pox and chicken pox, virus pneumonia and psittacosis, herpes zoster and poliomyelitis; in animals,
distemper in dogs, myxomatosis in rabbits, foot-and-mouth
disease in animals of cloven hoof. Viruses differ fundamentally
from the bacteria. They are much smaller, and now known to
consist of molecules of D.N.A. surrounded by an envelope of
protein, looking, under the electron microscope, rather like
doughnuts with the jam in the middle. They cannot reproduce
outside the body, but once in it, rapidly get into the cells to
which they are specific. There they penetrate the nucleus, and
start reproducing, interfering in the process with the normal
function of that cell. Hence the symptoms of the disease with
which they are associated. Whether a virus is alive or not depends on the definition of life adopted, if, indeed, life can any
longer be defined. Nevertheless, the reactions of the body
usually manage to overcome them, and, as the result of infection,
it usually develops immunity to re-infection. Almost everyone
recovers from mumps, measles, german measles and chicken
pox, and never gets them again. Small pox is a more serious
proposition, and poliomyeltis tends to leave permananet paralysis behind. But there are many different strains of the influenza

virus, and many of foot-and-mouth disease. This accounts for the fact that people do not get immune to 'flu, and explains why foot-and-mouth disease is so difficult to control.

Allergy

Immunity to infection depends on the fact that the body develops in such a way that the protein in bacteria and viruses stimulates the production in it of specific antibodies which tend to destroy the protein (i.e. the antigen), or react with it in such a way as to render it innocuous. But this property takes time to develop, and the body may be overwhelmed in the meantime by the intensity of the infection—in diphtheria or typhoid, for example—before its protective reactions have gathered sufficient strength. But, if the body survives, it has learnt something. It has learned to produce antibody, and its production is maintained with the result that it is now armed against reinfection, and in consequence, as we have just seen, is most unlikely to get that disease again.

This antigenic property in respect of the body is not a monopoly of bacterial and virus protein however. Rather, it is a general property of all protein, and in point of fact many proteins are always getting into us. A little escapes digestion, and gets through the mucous membrane of the gut. The emanations of animals, notably horses, dogs and cats, carry protein which gets into our systems through our lungs. Vegetable protein floats about in the air in the form of dusts, and in pollens in the spring and early summer, and these get into us through the mucous membrane of our noses and our conjunctivae. We live in fact in a protein environment, and the antigen-antibody structure of a man must in consequence be exceedingly complex.

Some people seem so made, for genetic or other reasons, that they are either deficient in the requisite antibodies to stand up to a certain antigen, or their antibodies to it are abnormal. This is known as allergy. Hence hay fever, which is certainly in part genetic—so often there is a history of it in the family—the antigen-antibody reaction taking place where the antigen gets in. Hence the swelling and congestion of the nose and eyes. Hence the bronchial spasm in asthma due to horses, and the gastro-intestinal attacks in people sensitive to shellfish or hen's eggs. The allergic state, too, is sometimes reflected in the skin. Nettle rash (urticaria) is a common manifestation of sensitivity.

The symptoms and course of many recognized bacterial infections are almost certainly in part allergic (i.e. due to reaction to antigen rather than to the direct action of the organisms on the body). This explains many of the clinical features of tuberculosis, and in some cases of tonsilitis—the streptococcus is the common cause of it—the disease starts a process known as specific rheumatism, characterized by joint pain and inflammation of the endocardium, the common cause of valvular disease of the heart in early life. In other cases it leads to acute inflammation of the kidneys, which can become chronic, leading to progressive renal failure, just as specific rheumatism can become chronic, leading to progressive heart failure.

Further, antigens can come from within as well as from without the body. For it is a community of cells serving different roles in the interest of it as a whole. The proteins of one cell are different to those of another. All are antigenic to the body as a whole, and all antigenic to it in different ways, demanding different antibodies to overcome them. Normally they are kept confined within cell membranes. Certain diseases, however, are associated with exposure to cold, malnutrition, emotional states, and the administration of certain drugs, and it is tempting to suppose that these tend to break down cell membranes, and that these diseases are auto-allergic in nature.

Two other diseases in particular may also prove allergic in this sense. One is rheumatoid arthritis, more prevalent in women than in men. This may occur at any age, but is more common in later adult life and characterized by progressive deformity and disintegration of the joints. (The heart is not affected as in specific rheumatism.) The other, which it is tempting to think about in these terms, is disseminated sclerosis. Again it is more common in women than men, but tends to occur in early adult life, and is characterized by patches of fibrosis scattered about in the nervous system. These lead to inco-ordination of speech and movement, and to progressive paralysis of upper motor neurone type.

The not-yet-understood

We do not know why so many infants are born with congenital

defects. Only a small proportion of them can be explained either in terms of inheritance or of chemical poisoning or infection during pregnancy.

We do not know why one organ sometimes seems to work too hard, at other times not hard enough, in relation to the requirements of the body as a whole. Why, for example, does the thyroid sometimes secrete too little thyroxine, leading to obesity, coarse skin and sterility (myxoedema); at other times too much, leading, because it sets the rate at which the machinery of the body ticks over at rest, to rapid loss of weight and, because it sensitizes the body to adrenaline, to nervousness (exopthalmic or toxic goitre)? Sometimes the bone marrow makes too little blood (aplastic anaemia). At other times it makes too much (polycythaemia).

We do not yet know why every now and then a person starts, and sometimes starts abruptly, to fail to use the glucose and non-nitrogenous part of the protein in his food, a process which depends on the secretion of insulin by his pancreas, leading, as would be expected, to rapid loss of weight, and compelling the excretion of sugar in the urine. (Although eating, he is in point of fact being starved.) Further, diabetes, as this condition is called, is not due, as might have been supposed, to simple failure of the pancreas to secrete enough insulin to meet the requirements of the body, comparable to thyroid failure in cretinism and myxoedmea. Rather, something seems to be antagonizing the action of it. A normal man requires about 20 units a day. A diabetic may demand 200.

We do not yet know why in many cases one or more of the constituents of the urine crystallize out in the kidneys, leading to stone formation, or why cholesterol may crystallize out in the gall bladder, leading to gall stones, predisposing to colic and biliary infection. We do not know why the mucous membrane of the stomach or duodenum sometimes gives way, leading to gastric or duodenal ulcer, or why some people develop ulceration of the colon. The cause of many skin diseases, psoriasis and lichen planus, for example, is still obscure. We can in fact describe diseases in terms of the structural changes in the body or the abnormal behaviour of it associated with them, give them names accordingly, list factors such as age, sex and circumstances with which they seem to be associated, and even treat them satisfactorily. But, excluding the infective diseases, the cause of most diseases still remains to a very large extent obscure. For no apparent reason, too, as age advances a man may develop cancer, or his blood pressure may rise dangerously, or he may die prematurely as the result of progressive arterial degeneration.

New growth

Sometimes certain cells, maybe a single cell in the first instance, instead of remaining respectable members of society in the niche to which they belong in the community of the body, start to divide and multiply out of all proportion to the requirements of it as a whole. This is known as neoplasia or new growth, although abnormal growth would have been a better term. All growth is new, and new in proportion to its age.

Some tumours produced in this way remain circumscribed, and are often surrounded by a capsule of fibrous tissue which the surrounding tissues have laid down in their defence. These may cause local symptoms by their unsightliness or by pressing on nerves or veins in their vicinity, and are said to be benign. Others start to infiltrate into the surrounding tissues, and then cells are carried away in the body fluids to give rise to secondary deposits elsewhere. These are said to be malignant, as untreated they are destined to destroy the body which gave birth to them. Indeed, if the community of cells which make it up is compared to an orderly society, malignant growth is a revolutionary attempt on the part of a certain group to usurp power resulting in the eventual destruction of the state.

Malignant growth is of two varieties. One originates in cells covering surfaces or lining hollow organs—the skin, the mucous membrane of the gut, the epethelium of the lungs—and is known as carcinoma. The other derives from solid organs, for example, bone, muscle, lymphatic gland, connective and blood-forming tissue, and is known as sarcoma, leukaemia—increase in the number of white cells in the blood—being a variety of it. Carcinoma tends to occur in later life. Sarcoma, which is much less common, may develop at any age. Both varieties are known to the laity as cancer.

The cause of malignant growth occurring naturally is not yet understood, but both types of this aberration of cell behaviour are known to be produced by over-exposure to ionizing radiation. Carcinoma occurs in X-ray burns. Leukaemia follows an atomic explosion and over-exposure to X-rays. Both can also be produced by the application of certain substances derived from coal tar. Painted on the skin these lead to carcinoma; injected, to carcinoma or sarcoma, depending on the tissue in which they land. Growths of this kind can be kept going indefinitely by transplantation from animal to animal without re-application of the carcinogen. Some types of sarcoma which occur in birds and animals can, however, be transmitted by the injection of cell-free extracts of them. This suggests that these are due to the action of something of a virus kind.

Two theories have been advanced to account for malignant growth.

According to one, this sudden acquisition of the habit of regardless division is due to the mutation of certain genes within the cell, leading to breakdown in the normal communicating machinery which exists between cells and controls their habits in relation to one another. In consequence it now starts to divide regardless of its neighbours and, as this defect is transmitted at each division, a colony of 'rogue' cells results. This concept fits the fact that mutation can be produced in insects by exposure to X-rays and by chemical means.

According to the second, malignant growth is due to the usurpation of cell government by a virus which gets in from outside and, having got in, replicates itself at each cell division so that it is passed on to the resulting daughter cells, and this new form of government perpetuated. This concept fits in with the fact that viruses are now known to be large self-reproducing molecules which get into cells and influence their habits.

The first of these theories seems to fit the facts relating to carcinoma, the second, many of those relating to sarcoma. But there are possible links between them, accounting perhaps for some of the intermediate types of malignant growth which are known to exist. Perhaps a virus can lead to mutation like a carcinogen. Or, it may be, a virus is to be regarded as a gene got loose, and that viruses are produced by carcinogens. For viruses are derived from cells, and are to be regarded as the product, rather than the precursors of them, as was thought at first.

But, even when the mechanism of the pathogenesis of cancer comes to be understood, when we know what mutates the genes or what leads a gene to get loose and become a virus, the problem of why one man gets cancer and another escapes, seems likely to remain. Certain aetiological facts are realized however. Cigarette smoking predisposes to cancer of the lung, although the actual carcinogen has not yet been identified. Skin cancer is produced by tar; carcinoma of the bladder by parasites. Age is a factor in the pathogenesis of carcinoma, particularly of carcinoma of the prostate. Nor can genetic factors be ruled out. Mice can be bred which all die of spontaneous cancer, and there are human families in which it appears in every generation. There are some in which every member seems destined to die of it, if he or she escapes the other risks to which human beings are exposed.

Blood pressure

Everyone must have some pressure in his arteries in order to remain alive. It is essential to get the blood up against gravity to the head, essential to get it round the body even when a man is lying down, and it is maintained in his large arteries by the output of his heart working against the resistance offered by his small ones. Call that off, and his blood pressure slumps and he faints. Call off the output of the heart, and again his pressure slumps and he faints. But in health a constant average pressure is maintained in the large arteries by the rapid adaptation of the resistance to the flow of blood to the rate of cardiac output, and by that of cardiac output to the amount of work in hand.

In some people the peripheral resistance to the flow of blood rises in later life due to spasm of the muscle in the walls of their small ateries, reducing their lumen and rendering it necessary for them to maintain a higher pressure in their large ones to get the blood through them. In fact, their disease, if so it can be called, is not their high blood pressure, but the constriction of their arterioles rendering that necessary. If their blood pressure under these circumstances did not rise, their circulation would fail. (The doctor does not try to get blood pressure down. Rather, he endeavours to relax arteriolar spasm.) But the consequences of it over a long period are inescapable. In the first place, as the heart has to work harder to maintain the circulation at rest, it has less reserve in hand when a greater circulation rate is needed. In consequence a man with high blood pressure gets unduly short of breath on exertion, and rapid rise of blood pressure, necessitated by sudden vaso-constriction (malignant hypertension), leads to acute heart failure. In the second, high blood pressure increases the mechanical strain to which the arteries are exposed, and, as would be expected, accelerates the degenerative process in them which is an invariable accompaniment of age.

Degeneration

A man is as old as his arteries. So runs the saying, and there is truth in it. The arteries tend to wear out more quickly in some men than in others, and always more quickly in men than women, a process accelerated by rise of blood pressure.

Arteriosclerosis, that is to say hardening and narrowing of arteries and roughening of their smooth internal lining, is essentially a patchy process. Some arteries are always more affected than others, and those most affected in one man may be the least affected in another. In the large ones it does not matter much. There is plenty of room for the blood to get past any obstruction. But narrowing of a small artery inevitably leads to gradual failure, and, if the blood clots in it, to sudden failure, of blood flow to the organ it supplies.

If one of the arteries to the heart gets narrower, although it can still carry enough blood when a man is resting, it cannot carry enough of it to enable him to hurry up a hill. So he is pulled up by pain in his chest. If the blood actually clots in it, and this may occur at any time, the blood supply to it is completely cut off, leading to severe pain. Coronary thrombosis is the common cause of sudden death.

If the arteries to the legs begin to narrow, a man is pulled up, after he has walked a certain distance, by pain in his calves, and compelled to rest before he can start again. If the blood clots in one of them, that leg goes white and numb and, unless the blood can reach his foot by some other route, gangrene, i.e. local death of tissue, due to failure of oxygen supply, starts in his toes and may involve his whole foot.

In the brain there are seldom any warnings of arterial disease, and the common consequence of cerebral arteriosclerosis is a sudden stroke. This may be due to thrombosis, as in a coronary attack, or to rupture of a vessel, cerebral haemorrhage, the arteries in the brain being peculiarly weak. The one supplying the tracts descending from the motor cortex is most often affected, and thrombosis and haemorrhage in the same place both lead to the same result. A man suddenly loses, or partially loses, consciousness with paralysis or paresis of the opposite side of his body, and when the left side of the brain is affected in a right-handed person, he also loses the power of speech.

Other parts of the body wear out for no other apparent reason than the passage of time and the stress of human existence. But genetic factors are really more important. There are short-lived and long-lived families, while identical twins, if they both escape all the risks to which human life is exposed, often die arterio-sclerotic deaths within a few months of each other. Indeed, a man's lease of life is largely determined at his conception, the quality of the stuff out of which he is made being more important than the care with which he drives his bodily machine.

In women the sexual cycle ceases round about the age of fifty. In men the climacteric is more gradual. In both sexes the hair turns grey, and the skin loses its elasticity and becomes wrinkled, adding character to the face. Degenerative changes in the lens lead to failing vision (cataract); in the ear, to increasing deafness (otosclerosis). They are also common in the lungs (emphysema), and in the weight-bearing joints (osteo-arthritis). The body usually fails before the mind. But sometimes the mind fails first. Lear, the classical case of senile dementia in literature, still looked to Kent, 'every inch the King'.

The psychosomatic concept

We still do not know the cause of many, if not most, diseases; and even when there would appear to be an obvious one, a chemical poison or a pathogenic bacillus, for instance, it is often difficult to explain why one man succumbed, but for some reason another, living under similar circumstances, escaped. Certainly, although we can sometimes recognize predisposing factors, we do not know why one man gets cancer, another develops high blood pressure, a third dies in a coronary attack. So it is often asked whether the mind developed on the body may not play some part in predisposing it to succumb to some of the known causes of disease, chemical poisoning and infection, for instance, and to the many of the diseases to which man is heir but are not yet understood. In fact, just as some diseases are somatopsychic in the sense that some peculiarity of body predisposes the mind to succumb to mental stress up to which most men can stand, may not some be psychosomatic, in the sense that some peculiarity of mind predisposes the body to succumb to physical factors which it would normally be able to resist? A man can, of course, deliberately run his body into risk. But can mental states, such as stress, anxiety, unhappiness, disappointment, lead him to succumb to one of the risks in life to which, in a happier or more settled state of mind, he would not have succumbed, or lead him to develop one of those strange diseases which have just been listed? Is high blood pressure, for example, due to stress in a person predisposed by his constitution to develop it? Is it possible for a man to die of a broken heart under certain circumstances? Could the news of Austerlitz, as the history books say, really have killed the younger Pitt?

In theory there is no reason why this should not happen. Every time a man wills any movement, a process at the conscious level of body-mind initiates chemical changes in certain muscles which lead them to swell up, that is to say, temporarily change their structure, with the result that they approximate their points of attachment and effect the movement willed. But there is clearly no dividing line between transient chemical, with transient structural change, and permanent chemical, with permanent structural change, the latter so often found in organic disease. In theory, too, it could happen. States of mind predispose to auto-allergic conditions, and physiology is narrowing the gap between mind and body. Emotional states are now known to be associated with the activity of centres in the brain stem, and these control the pituitary which lies in close connection with them. This in turn, by virtue of its hormones, regulates the activity of all the other endocrines, including the cortex of the adrenal glands. This secretes cortisone which regulates the reaction of the body to stress, injury and infection.*

Neurotic people seem to be no more liable to organic disease than stable people. Some, perhaps, are less so. Their way of life protects them. Clinical experience, on the other hand, suggests, not only that certain diseases tend to follow nervous shock or to be associated with mental stress, but that they are also associated with the way in which body-mind has developed. Personality predisposes to them. This statement seems true of thyrotoxicosis, ulcerative colitis, asthma, and many skin diseases. Further, doctors see cardiac infarction, malignant hypertension, cancer, follow stress more often than many are prepared to write off as pure coincidence. Therefore, although organic disease may never be entirely psychogenic, some seem so constituted that they are liable to develop a certain kind of it when subjected to stress, while others, made of sterner stuff, can stand up to any amount of it.

In the present state of medical knowledge it is, however, unwise to over-rate the importance of mental states in the pathogenesis of organic disease. Somatic causes of it, besides those already recognized, may lie just round the corner. Microorganisms were recognized as a cause of it less than a hundred years ago. Ionizing radiation is a still more recent discovery. Before long we shall have found out much more about the influence of genetic factors in the pathogenesis of it, and perhaps discover chemical risks in the soil of which we remain completely unaware at present. But few diseases, it seems, are likely to be due to single causes. Physical injury and chemical poisoning are often the result of the interaction of many factors, genetic, traumatic, infective, psychological, and the aetiology of those as yet little understood is likely to be even more complex. Many can in fact probably compare to thunderstorms, in the sense that the right concatination of circumstances is needed. To get them a man must be of a certain psychosomatic constitution, and collide at a certain age with certain adverse factors at a time when he is

---

* In these conditions the body steps up the secretion of cortisone, and for this reason little is gained by giving it, unless a patient is known to be deficient in the secretion of it. Then he is usually on cortisone already, and under these circumstances his dose is immediately increased.

emotionally upset or under stress, and for some reason his health is depressed.

So, in these days attempts are being made, both in the armed forces and in industry, to assess men as fit or unfit in relation to what is likely to be demanded of them. They are classed according to physical make-up, bodily architecture, muscular development, staying power, habits and characteristics, particularly the tendency to put on weight and disinclination to take exercise both known to predispose to hypertension and coronary disease. They are also assessed from the point of view of mental qualities, intelligence, courage, capacity for leadership, reaction to responsibility, and the strength of their personality. To some extent, too, we can now put the physical and the psychological together. We are beginning to recognize the type of man who will break down physically under emotional stress.

On the other hand, men still get strange and weird diseases for which no psychosomatic predisposition, no physical cause nor any emotional experience can account at present. These must possess some genetic defect, or for some reason their defence mechanisms break down, or an unpredictable molecular accident leads to mutation, altering the behaviour of certain cells, or somatic or psychological causes of diseases exist of which we can take no account as yet. So, in the assessment of risk in relation to constitution, doctors must not over-call their hands. But the day does seem to be approaching when it should become possible to survey a man, and find out whether his health is founded on a rock or whether, like the house in the parable, in spite of its imposing appearance, it is really built upon the sand.

*   *   *

Organic disease is faulty development of, or adverse action on, the body stimulating reactions which tend to maintain life and restore order, the two, action and reaction, conspiring to lead to the symptoms of which a person complains. Sometimes his symptoms are mainly due to action on his body; at other times mainly due to reaction by it. In either case he thinks he has 'got something'. For we tend to think of diseases as things which overtake us. Their names and talk about cases of this or that suggest it. The description of them rubs in this idea. And yet, as a moment's thought reveals, diseases no more exist apart from people than battles exist when they are not being fought, although, just as we can talk about battles of a certain kind, so we can talk about diseases of a certain kind. A disease is an abstract concept. It cannot exist without a man to suffer from it any more than a human mind can exist without a human body to maintain it.

A disease is an alteration in a person for the worse, and, while it lasts, he is physically and emotionally mal-adapted to his environment. Further, disease creates a problem, not only for the man himself, but also for other people. Only in very exceptional circumstances is he ill in splendid isolation. Far more often someone else must do his work. Someone else may have to continue theirs, and at the same time look after him. His illness may lead to anxiety in his family. It may be infectious. It may be serious. He may be dying. It may precipitate neurotic or emotional reactions in other people. In short a sick man influences his environment profoundly. Further, he creates a problem for his doctor, and disease in general, both functional and organic, creates a problem for society incorporated into the State.

CHAPTER VIII

HEALTH, SOCIETY, LAW

*Eating—Smoking—Drinking—Drugs—Sex—Termination
—Sterilization—Marriage, children and divorce—Compulsory restraint.*

In a modern society, particularly in one which maintains a
health service available to all, part of a man's duty, it can be
argued, is to keep as fit as his constitution and circumstances
permit in order to make his contribution to society and avoid
becoming a burden on it. Further, not only does every man
create an environment for himself, which may be beneficial or
prejudicial to his own health, but he also consciously or unconsciously helps to create an environment beneficial or prejudicial
to that of other people. Human health also depends on personal
relationships. A man should not offend against either the environment or person of other men. So society incorporated into
the state passes Acts of Parliament from time to time in order to
modify or limit common law, or amend statute law, in such a
way as to ensure a healthy environment and maintain right
human relationships in the light of changing public opinion and
new discoveries. These protect the individual from himself and
from society, and society from the individual. But matters of this
kind often necessitate restriction of individual liberty, and the
Churches would have all laws conform to principles based on
Christianity. Acts of Parliament relating to them are often only
passed by majority decisions in both Houses.*

* Common law, the customary law of England dating from the reign of
Richard II or earlier, has been modified in its application again and again
by the creation of statute law by Act of Parliament. The common law of
England differs from the common law of Scotland, but common law is
largely peculiar to this country. The legal system of most others is based on
codes of law.

Eating

Man, like every other animal, must eat to live, and a daily minimum of protein is essential to the maintenance of his health. So whenever food is short, individual consumption is restricted so that everyone gets a fair share, as in the rationing systems in operation during both world wars. In time of peace no restriction of liberty in this respect is necessary, and except in the lowest income groups, which are now provided for by the State, eating is often dictated by pleasure rather than necessity. In consequence in an affluent society many eat too much in relation to the work they do, predisposing to obesity and coronary disease. Further, a certain amount of physical exertion would also appear to be necessary to health, although instinct does not dictate it, at least not in adult life. Rather, mechanical devices in developed countries, by removing the necessity to exert the body, combined with the temptation to eat too much—wild animals work for their food and live hungry—has added a new risk to life, to which some would appear to succumb.

Smoking

Smoking is a habit deeply rooted in the lives of many men, a habit, too, which is a considerable source of revenue to the State. But cigarette smoking particularly is now known to predispose to coronary disease, bronchitis and lung cancer. Most men and women are still dragged into it, however, and live exposed to these risks.

Some therefore, putting the health of society before personal liberty, would have the government tax cigarette smoking out of existence. Others, putting personal liberty before the health of society, maintain that it must not be taxed up to this point. A man has the right to take any risk he likes provided it does not interfere with anybody else. But most would have the government continue to steer the pragmatic course which it adopts at present. Everything possible should be done to dissuade people from starting a habit which so easily comes to exceed the bounds of self-control. They would prohibit advertising different brands and the augmentation of sales by coupon devices. But they would not prevent cigarette smoking altogether. In moderation it suits some, and does little harm to others; and the fact remains that the abolition of it by excessive taxation would be a source of embarrassment to the exchequer. This position is, of of course, morally, financially, and medically unsatisfactory. The problem can be solved only by the production of a carcino-gen-free cigarette.

Drinking

Alcohol releases inhibition and engenders cheerfulness. Whether it actually reduces reaction-times and makes for quicker think-ing, is doubtful, although in the popular mind it is regarded as a stimulant. What is certain is that it takes the edge off reality, and oils the wheels of human life.

Most people learn to drink in moderation, and on this scale alcohol does little physical or mental harm. In the West it has become part of the way of life of most men and many women. Alcohol is paraded on every great occasion. The only attempt in fact made to control its consumption is by licensing public houses, restricting opening hours, and forbidding the sale of alcoholic drinks to children. Further, although first taxed in the eighteenth century, when the gin laws were passed in order to control a fast growing social evil ('Drunk for a penny, dead drunk for twopence'), ever since duty has been levied on it more with the idea of raising revenue—and it has never been taxed too high—than with any intention of preventing drunkenness.

Recently the problem assumed new proportions. A small con-centration of alcohol in the blood materially interferes with co-ordination between eye and hand, and any man who drinks, and then drives, is acting irresponsibly in relation to his own life, the lives of his passengers, and those of other people on the road. The individual risk is, of course, small, and for this reason many are content to take it with the result that accidents due to this cause add up to a high proportion of the total mortality of the roads. The problem is how to try to stop people taking it beyond a certain point. Publicity had failed, and society would hardly stand for prohibition. That has never lasted long in any country, and it would mean a heavy loss of revenue which could only be made good by a considerable increase in direct taxation. So com-pulsory tests for alcohol in the blood of drivers of motor vehicles in certain circumstances have been introduced at the expense of some infringement of individual liberty.

Others became addicted to alcohol in the sense that they are now dependent on the regular consumption of large quantities, and cannot give it up. This may be the result of opportunity or circumstances. A man can afford it. The nature of his work forces him into it. Or his will may be weak; he starts it, and then cannot stop. The craving gets too great. Another takes to it as a way of escape from reality. But, whatever the cause of addiction, the consumption of large quantities over long periods leads to progressive deterioration in body and mind, partly due to the direct action on the body and partly due to neglect of personal health. In one man, progressive mental deterioration dominates the scene; in another, cirrhosis of the liver, or failure of the peripheral nerves due to vitamin B deficiency born of dietetic neglect. Further, any acute infection, or sudden deprivation of the alcohol to which the body has become accustomed, may precipitate an attack of acute excitement (derlirium tremens). A wage packet spent on drink leads of necessity to poverty and to all its social consequences.

Drugs

A drug is any substance used in medicine, but the word now implies in the lay mind something that a person takes with the object of altering his mood. In this sense alcohol is very much a drug, although it has become so much a part of many people's way of life that few think of it as such. Some drugs reduce pain (analgesics). Others promote sleep (hypnotics). Some calm the mind (tranquillizers). Others counter depression (anti-depressants). All these, and many others, are dangerous to the health of the body, and their sale and distribution are controlled by the Pharmacy and Poisons Act under which they can be obtained only on a doctor's prescription. But the ones people ordinarily mean when they talk of drugs are those which stimulate a man into action, increase pleasure, detach him from reality, or lead to hallucinations. These are also dangerous to the health of the mind, in the sense that a person can become so dependent on them that he cannot give them up or is unable to give them up without withdrawal symptoms. Further, some lead to progres-

sive mental and moral deterioration. Their manufacture is therefore controlled by the Dangerous Drugs Act which also imple-
ments certain international conventions to which the United
Kingdom is party. Had alcohol been discovered yesterday, it
would probably have been controlled by it too.

Marajuana, or cannabis resin, one of the most ancient of drugs,
usually smoked in cigarettes (reefers), leads to detachment from
reality and hallucinations which take the form of exaggeration of
normal experience. While alcohol tends to extroversion, rendering it easier for a shy person to get on with other people, cannabis
turns a man's mind in upon himself. In the Middle East it has
long found its place in society as alcohol has found its place in the
West. While in the latter it is respectable to drink alcohol, and
disreputable to smoke cannabis, in the former the converse holds.
Some maintain that, in view of the difficulty in controlling the
sale of cannabis on the black market, it should be struck off the
list of drugs controlled by law, and allowed to find its place in
society—as alcohol has long since done—backing up this view
with the argument that it is always tempting to try out the for-
bidden. Some go further. They question the right of society to
interfere with personal liberty. Those who want to smoke cannabis should be free to enjoy it. Others argue against decontrol.
Cannabis, although it has little effect on personality, leads to
disorientation. Driving a car or riding a motor cycle under it is
dangerous, and there is no test for it in the blood to facilitate
convictions. The problem created by alcohol is great enough
without another one added to it. Further, many believe that
addicts to 'soft' drugs run some risk of escalating into addiction
to 'hard' ones, cannabis sometimes being labelled, in popular
terminology, 'soft' as opposed to morphine, heroin and cocaine,
which are called 'hard'.

Opium eating and smoking are of great antiquity, and morphine has long been used in medicine. A number of synthetic
compounds allied to morphine are also now extant, and heroin,
a derivative of it, has an even more engaging effect on the
human mind, engendering a dreamy state and detachment from
reality. To become an addict to heroin is easy. Dependence on it
is soon absolute. It also leads, more rapidly even than morphine,
to progessive deterioration.

The mental stimulants are few and far between. Alcohol is, as we have already seen, a doubtful starter. The only real ones are caffein, the active constituent of tea and coffee, the amphetamines and cocaine. The action of the former is well known. The amphetamines heighten awareness, and help a person to keep awake. They can cause mild hallucinations, and have led to irresponsible behaviour. They also lead to strange consequences when taken by candidates before examinations. Their distribution and sale is not controlled by the Dangerous Drugs Act, and although they are on the Poisons List, and should only be obtainable on prescription, adolescents have little difficulty in getting hold of 'purple hearts' of which an amphetamine is the main constituent. Cocaine acts as an immediate, almost lightning stimulant and increases all forms of physical pleasure, that is to say, as long as its action lasts. The reaction afterwards is severe, and addiction to it is even more difficult to break than addiction to heroin.

A number of drugs have been recently produced, notably L.S.D. and S.T.P., which tend to produce hallucinations, much like those which occur naturally in psychotic states. Sometimes these are terrifying or even dangerous. A man has stepped out of a third-floor window confident that he could walk on air. They can also lead to serious depression. What place, if any, they have in medicine is at present uncertain, but they are only administered under strict supervision. So, although they do not seem habit-forming, if, as is generally conceded, it is the duty of the State to protect the public against traumatic risks and accidental poisoning, it is equally its duty to protect people against these dangers at the price of some restriction of liberty. No one is now allowed to experiment in these drugs for fun.

Until comparatively recently drug addiction in the U.K. was mainly confined to adults who had been put on a drug for medical reasons in the first instance. During the last ten years or so it has, as everyone knows, assumed unprecedented proportions, and worked its way down into colleges and universities and even into schools. Drug-taking has become an adolescent fashion. Many reasons have been assigned for this development. At all ages it provides escape from reality. In young adults, too much money often conspires with nothing particular to do, lack of a sense of responsibility and emotional instability; in the teenage group, lack of parental authority and the decline of religious teaching with the pressure of examinations, often against an unhappy home background. Moreover, there is always fun in a new experience and an element of bravado in it. If the leader of a gang or group takes drugs, the others must start to do so also, and there is prestige in the possession of a syringe. All the talk about drugs in the press and on television also puts ideas into heads. Many would never have started taking drugs, had they not heard so much about them.

In the eighteenth and nineteenth centuries opium, and later morphine, were the drugs most taken. Laudanum, tincture of opium, was much used in medical practice, particularly in the treatment of consumption, and de Quincey, was, of course, an opium eater. Injecting oneself with morphine came in later, as syringes were perfected, but injecting oneself with cocaine only became a serious form of addiction in the thirties. Now the 'hard' drug usually taken is heroin, often combined with cocaine, both leading to progressive deterioration. The addict becomes increasingly slovenly in his habits, more and more irresponsible at his work, and before long to all intents and purposes unemployable. For drug addiction becomes a full-time occupation, an addict living for his next shot, and often neglecting his general health in consequence, his expectation of life now seriously curtailed. Some die of an over-dose; others of virus hepatitis, or septic poisoning contracted as the result of contaminated syringes. Many manage to become experts at injecting themselves intravenously which, both from the point of view of infection and also from that of over-dose, is peculiarly dangerous.

Drug addiction can be tackled in two ways. Drugs might be rendered virtually unobtainable. This was the policy behind the Dangerous Drugs Act in 1923, but was in part defeated by illicit traffic in them. Further, addicts can seldom be cured, or anyhow have seldom been cured in the past, and yet the symptoms of withholding a drug to which the body has become habituated can be very severe. So doctors were forced into prescribing drugs for addicts who often persuaded them to give them more than they really wanted. Or they would 'lose' their prescriptions, and come back for another. Or they would steal prescription forms, and forge their doctor's signature. Some doctors, too, were lax in their prescribing habits. In short, medical prescribing was found to be the main source of drugs on the black market in this country, and the law has been amended to deal with this situation.

Under the Dangerous Drugs Act of 1967 a doctor can now only prescribe heroin or cocaine for medical purposes; to relieve pain, for example, or to ease the passage of a dying man. Further, he is now under an obligation to notify an addict to either of these drugs in his practice to the Home Office, and his patient is then referred to one of the special treatment centres now established. There he is kept supplied with his drug instead of obtaining it under false pretences or on the black market. Addicts are no longer tempted or forced into peddling some of their drugs at a high price in order to afford to buy more of it for themselves. At least that is the theory, and by this method it is hoped to reduce the demand for these drugs, and defeat the illicit trade in them. How well this Act which at present only deals with two drugs, namely, heroin and cocaine, is working out in practice, and how successful the new centres will prove in curing addiction, the future will reveal.

The other way of tackling this problem is health education. Alcohol, some would say, sets an unfortunate example. But an effort is now being made to encourage adolescents to build into their personalities a natural resistance to interfering with the machinery of the brain by taking drugs. The psychosomatic concept and the idea of the value of personal integrity in relation to society are both essential to health education.

Sex

The traditional standards and values relating to human conduct still mostly hold good as ideals. Indeed, only in one department of it has secular opinion changed radically, namely, in that relating to sex, the austere concept of sexuality as sin which obscures spiritual vision and celibacy and virginity as the most exalted states, having largely given place to the concept of sexuality as natural, and sexual life necessary for most people.

Further, the material deterrent to irregularity in sex relationships, namely illegitimate pregnancy, has been largely eliminated of recent years. Male contraceptives have long been easily available, and contraceptive clinics for women have been in operation for some time. The latter were first started by voluntary effort. Now they are maintained by local authorities, and unmarried women of all ages, if they want help in this direction, are encouraged to attend. Conception can also now be prevented, not only by mechanical, but also by chemical means. For the hormone produced during pregnancy, calling off the sexual cycle, can be taken at will to prevent ovulation. Many doctors hesitate to prescribe chemical contraceptives for long periods however, particularly to young women. There is little immediate danger in taking them, but they suppress a normal function, and the long-term consequences of that cannot be foreseen. They are not the ideal contraceptive. That would be something which prevented male and female germ cells from fusing, rather than stopping them meeting, or inhibiting their production.*

The Roman Catholic Church, in spite of these developments, in spite of over-population in relation to food supply in many countries, in spite of considerable pressure from its own laity, puts spiritual values before material things, and has recently in a Papal Encyclical reaffirmed its objection to the use of contraceptives of any kind whatever, a decision which has precipitated a wide division of opinion within the Roman Church, some of its adherents now claiming the right to act as conscience dictates. But the doctrine stands: to prevent conception is to cheat God's purpose and to sin. So the only methods of family planning open to Roman Catholics are abstinence and the safe period, their church maintaining a distinction between the sexual act performed, knowing that pregnancy is unlikely to result for natural reasons, and the taking of deliberate steps to prevent it at a time when the sexual act would otherwise lead to it. Roman Catholics therefore tend to have larger families, and families larger than they can support, more often than members of other Christian denominations, and Catholic

* A chemical contraceptive has been recently discovered which acts by preventing the fertilized ovum from becoming embedded in the uterine mucous membrane, and would appear to be effective even if taken after intercourse. It has not yet been released for distribution.

countries run a greater risk of over-population in relation to food supply than others, a situation justified by the belief that the misery of this world is unimportant in view of the nature of the world to come and the purpose of creation.

Right-wing Anglican opinion also maintains that, for some at least, the austerity of the celibate life widens spiritual vision. But all Christian denominations, other than Roman Catholicism, hold that for ordinary people the sexual act within monogamous marriage (by mutual consent) is of value in promoting right relationships in married life. So, although they deplore deliberate childlessness, and look upon it as selfish, contravening the purpose for which marriage was ordained, they allow family planning by means of contraceptives in relation to physical health and the situation in which parents are placed. Families within these denominations tend to be smaller. The unwanted child within marriage is also less common, and a non-Catholic country runs less risk of over-population in relation to food supply. Further, holding that intercourse without the intent to procreate is permissible within marriage, they are beginning to look with increasing tolerance on intercourse outside it when, for some reason, marriage is impossible but love and companionship exist. The World Council of Churches recently conceded that pre-marital sexual intercourse is permissible in certain circumstances.

Secular opinion approaches the problem from the point of view of biological fact unfettered by the concept of sin. There is no harm in indulgence in moderation unless it mars the life of the other partner to the act, leads to an unwanted child (for which there is little excuse in view of the availability and efficiency of modern contraceptives), interferes with development or leads to deterioration of personality by using energy which could have been directed into other channels, or leads to sense of guilt when by it a man offends against his own conscience, predisposing him to neurotic breakdown. Nevertheless, fidelity is held the social ideal in most secular circles, promiscuity being clearly an offence against personal integrity in relation to society, as evidenced in the latter by prostitution, venereal disease and illegitimacy. Every man should, both in the interest of his own self-development, and in the interest of the maintenance of the health and happiness of the greatest number, endeavour to maintain his own personal integrity in matters relating to sex. Many fall far short of this ideal. But to depart from faith in it as such, as already pointed out (p. 88), predisposes to neurosis, leading to mal-adaptation to circumstances. Failure to see the necessity for it is a manifestation of the social regardlessness of the psychopathic mind.

The use of contraceptives is a decision for the individual rather than the doctor, but the latter is often asked to advise on contraceptive technique and the prescription of chemical contraceptives is vested in his hands. Personal and emotional problems are often found to be involved, and they cannot be doled out regardless. For instance, should a possible or potential prostitute be put on the pill? There are risks both ways; destruction of personal integrity at the expense of society, on the one hand; the unwanted illegitimate child, on the other. When one doctor won't, there is often another who will. But in each case right action depends on whether anything can be done to restore sense of personal integrity in relation to society, or alter the circumstances in which the individual is placed.

Termination

Abortion cannot be induced with any certainty by medical means, and is only attempted at some risk. But pregnancy can be terminated surgically with only slight risk up to the end of the third month or a little later. (After that the uterus must be removed.) This is also known popularly as 'abortion' and, in view of the risk of infection in inexperienced hands, and the stand taken by the Churches on the moral issue at stake, it has long been controlled by law.

The Roman Catholic Church has resisted the legalization of the termination of pregnancy for some time. Just as it remains opposed to preventing conception, and depriving God of a new human soul, so it remains opposed to depriving a new human soul of the vehicle on which it is embarked on its journey through life. For, according to Roman Catholic theology, the soul enters the body at the moment of conception. So the Roman Catholic doctor must never induce abortion except to save the life of the mother when, of course, the child must also die, if he does not. In the later months of pregnancy, when the child becomes viable (i.e. capable of independent existence), he must put the life of the child before that of the mother.

Most religious people outside the Roman Catholic Church look upon the soul as something developed in, or acquired by, the body during late ante-natal or early post-natal life, and destined in some way to survive the death of it. Indeed, the view of many, whether reached subconsciously or actually thought out, does not differ materially from the scientific concept of the mind developing on, and conditioned by, the body as the result of the experience of living. Many remain doubtful whether the unborn child really has much soul. In fact the only real difference between the religious and agnostic points of view would often appear to be that, while the religious man, as a matter of faith, believes that the soul developed during life will survive the death of the body, the agnostic does not see how this can be on the evidence available.

Many outside the Churches approach the problem, as they approach that of contraception, free of preconceived ideas. Nature is prodigal. One pregnancy is as good as another, and all conceptions late in the ovarian cycle end naturally in unrecognized abortion. To them the unwanted child is the great evil, termination the last resort in birth control. But it is a clumsy method, and secular opinion admits that there is much to be said against free abortion apart from the religious and moral issues at stake. It is not without some risk. It demands admission to hospital, and that costs money; and why should the State pay for the termination of pregnancies resulting from careless living in respect of the much simpler and now easily available methods of birth control? Thirdly, a child unwanted before birth may prove much loved after birth. Fourthly, abortion, the deliberate destruction, as the result of a woman's own wish, or perhaps by her grudging consent, of a new unit of human life developing within her may have psychological consequences. Cases are on record in which she has never recovered her mental poise. Unrestricted abortion would encourage a degree of irresponsibility which could hardly be tolerated.

Until recently pregnancy could only be terminated legally if a woman's health, either physical or mental, would suffer as the result of it continuing. It could not be terminated because her pregnancy was the result of rape, or there was a strong probability that her child would be born abnormal. Nor could it be terminated merely because she would not be in a position to look after it properly, because it was illegitimate or unwanted, or because she thought she had enough children already. The concept of health was often stretched wide, but illegal abortion remained common, and, until antibiotics were introduced, the mortality of it remained high.

Under the Act of 1967 the termination of pregnancy is now legal if, in the opinion of any two doctors, there is reasonable probability that the child will be born in some way abnormal. Further, under the Act's social clauses the environment into which the child will be born, its mother's ability to bring it up properly, and the interests of her other children, can all be taken into account. But illegitimacy, except in so far as the birth of an illegitimate child may affect a woman's mental health, does not constitute grounds for termination under the new any more than it did under the old law, and the clause in the Bill legalizing termination of pregnancy resulting from a sexual offence was deleted during its passage through Parliament.

Many difficulties seem likely to arise under the new law. How great must be the chance of a child being born abnormal to justify termination? Further, if the degree of probability required can be agreed, how is it to be assessed in the individual case? How late in pregnancy, for instance, does german measles constitute a serious risk of malformation? Medical knowledge is not yet sufficient to give the definite answers which the law appears to demand.

The social clauses are also bound to create difficulties. Whether a woman's circumstances, or the interests of her other children, justify abortion will often be hard to decide, and on any standards there are bound to be differences of opinion in this matter. Further, the same wide range of opinion on the ethics of abortion as exists among the laity also exists within the medical profession. Some doctors remain opposed to the new law on conscientious grounds, and will either refuse to implement it or interpret its permissive provisions strictly. The evidence for german measles will need to be convincing, and it will have to have occured early in pregnancy. The woman's circumstances will have to be deplorable, or her family large already. Those on the left, who hold that abortion ought to be easily available to women who want it, will, on the other hand, accept evidence for german measles without much question, and interpret the social provisions of the Act more liberally. So, if a woman's own doctors will not agree to terminate her pregnancy, she will not have much difficulty in finding two who will. While under the old law it was often difficult to justify abortion as legal, under the new law it will be difficult to prove it to have been illegal.

Practical difficulties seem also likely to arise. Pregnancy can still only be terminated surgically, and in involves admission to hospital. So again and again a doctor in a hard-pressed gynaecological unit will have to choose between taking in a woman for termination and a patient on the list to come in for, say, an operation for cancer of the cervix. Both are urgent. Time will show how things work out, but it seems likely that doctors with a tendency to interpret the law liberally, will use existing or even start new private nursing homes for this purpose. Under the Act these must be licensed by the Minister.

Sterilization

Sterilization, which renders it impossible for a woman to have, or a man to beget, children, or renders it impossible for a woman to have or a man to beget another, must also be regarded as a method of birth control. It can be effected either by removing the glands or exposing them to ionizing radiation or by tying the genital ducts. The former takes away the internal secretion of the gonads, and leads to failure of development or to regression, according to age, of the secondary sexual characteristics. It has been used from time immemorial in the East to produce eunuchs. It was used in Hitler's Germany in his attempt to destroy the Jewish race. In medical practice the latter method is always employed, permanent sterilization being easily effected by tying each Fallopian tube or vas. This does not lead to any psychosomatic change.

Sterilization is an offence against personal integrity, but it is a realistic way of handling the threat of population overtaking food supply in countries where the general level of education does not permit adequate control of birth by other methods. In

India, for instance, it is officially encouraged, but in this country it is illegal, as it necessitates an open operation, unless it can be justified on the grounds of necessity. For all surgery, it must be remembered, is by common law and by the Act of 1861 in fact a crime, an assault on the body, whether or not the patient has given his consent, and only justified in law by the fact that a greater evil has been averted. That of death from appendicitis, for example, or the continued risk associated with a duodenal ulcer, is greater than the evil committed, that is to say, incision into the abdomen and mutilation of internal parts.

Sterilization of a woman is only strictly legal if it would be dangerous for her to have children or harmful for her to have further children, an argument for it that is loosely used. Many women are now sterilized when they have had as many children as they want. Performed merely to prevent pregnancy in a woman without children, that is to say, as a method of birth control without medical justification, it would probably be found illegal if a case of this kind were ever brought to court. Any operation on a man merely to render him incapable of procreation might well be found illegal too, and if it is dangerous for a married woman to have children or to have another child, she must be sterilized, if need be, and not her husband. She might die, and he might marry again. Nor is sterilization really legal in either sex because some hereditary disease runs in one family, and husband and wife are anxious not to transmit it to their children. Easier methods of preventing birth are available. Further, pregnancy under these circumstances now constitutes legal grounds for termination.

Sterilization of sexual offenders has been employed in the Scandinavian countries, but is difficult to justify on moral grounds, and is clearly open to abuse. Large doses of ovarian hormone reduce the output of male hormone temporarily, however, decrease sex urge, and render the individual less liable to commit antisocial acts. Voluntarily accepted this can be justified on the grounds that it restores personal integrity in relation to society.

Marriage, children and divorce

The sexual instinct, psychosomatically engendered, combined

with desire for lifelong companionship, romanticized in literature and reinforced by tradition, urges the majority of people eventually to marry.

In most adolescents psychosexual development, after a brief homosexual phase, gives way to heterosexual interest, but no absolute dividing line can be drawn between homosexuality and heterosexuality, and the ratio of interest in these two directions varies to some extent with age. Some, however, grow up largely, or almost exclusively, homosexual in nature, although it does not follow that they indulge in homosexual practices. (Homosexuality and homosexual acts are not to be confused.) In the West the former has long been regarded as a perversion, something of which an individual ought to be ashamed—rather than as a misfortune for which he cannot be held responsible—and the latter by the Christian Churches as sin. In consequence in many countries homosexual acts were at one time, or still are, punishable by law, an attitude which, although it has protected the young, has led, or still leads, to much unhappiness. Homosexuality is not an uncommon cause both of neurotic breakdown and of serious depression. Recently a more liberal attitude in this matter has come to prevail in this country, and the Anglican Church, as opposed to the Roman and some of the dissenting denominations, has been in the vanguard of reform. Many, however, still see homosexuality as a menace to society, dominating, it is said, certain trades and professions, and forcing people into it. These opposed recent liberalization of the law as likely to lead to weakening of the public attitude toward homosexuality. But, except in the armed forces and merchant navy, a homosexual act between consenting adults in private under the Act of 1967 is no longer an offence.

But most people develop heterosexual, and in spite of the diffuse instinct of men (as opposed to the more possessive instinct of women), the Christian religion, the relatively equitable distribution of wealth, and the approximate numerical equality of the sexes, have conspired in the West to lead to monogamous marriage as the accepted custom. The absence of a breeding season in man also dictates a mate for life. This ideal has in fact followed in the wake of biological necessity, and as such was adopted by the Church. Casual relationships are a departure from the social as well as from the religious ideal.

The fact that in man sexual maturity ante-dates physical maturity, when childbirth becomes safe, and marriage is legal complicates the problem of the choice of mate. The fact that mental maturity is still longer delayed complicates it further. Again and again this choice is made, under the urge of instinct, by a mind still immature, and the risk is that sexual interest is romanticized into the false conviction that he or she will provide all that is wanted by the mind. In consequence mistakes are made, and the foundation of many unhappy marriages laid at the time they are undertaken. Others grow apart, as personality develops further, and many marriages break down, often with disastrous consequences both to the health and happiness of the children of them.

Extreme views, quite apart from religious considerations, are taken in the matter of divorce. Some, thinking of the health and happiness of the children, would have it difficult to get. Others, thinking of the position in which parents may be placed, would grant it on grounds of incompatibility of temperament. In practice the law relating to the annulment of civil marriage compromises between these points of view. But the fact remains that while the former, the traditional and clerical, is based on biological fact, the latter derives from modern sentiment. The unity of family life in the interest of health must be maintained, it can be argued, regardless of personal cost. The health of society, which is the health of all its members, depends very largely on it. Some, of course, attempting to forecast the future, have questioned whether, if present trends continue, the institution of marriage will survive. But it holds the field at present, and the family remains the unit of society.

Childlessness in marriage is sometimes deliberate but far more often due to psychological factors. In most cases these are amenable to treatment and, if normal relationships cannot be established, a woman can usually be artificially inseminated by her own husband, A.I.H. In other cases a marriage remains childless, either for no apparent reason, or because a husband cannot inseminate his wife—nor can she be artificially inseminated by him—on account of disease having blocked his genital ducts. Under the former circumstances the woman might, and under the latter probably would, become pregnant as the result of intercourse with another man. But this would be adultery, and, unless she obtained her husband's consent, would render her liable to be divorced. Further, if the paternity of the child could be established, it might be ruled illegitimate. Under both circumstances artificial insemination by an anonymous donor (A.I.D.) is sometimes practised. If the woman keeps this secret from her husband, he thinks that he is the father of the child. If he finds out, and could prove his case, he could probably get a divorce on grounds of adultery. If he could prove that the child was not by him, he would establish its illegitimacy and loss of right to inherit.

In the vast majority of cases A.I.D. is practised by mutual consent on the part of a childless couple, and remains a well-guarded secret between husband, wife and doctor. Nor, unless husband-wife relationships break down, is the child ever likely to come to know that it is not born of both its parents, and it will certainly be regarded by relations and friends as legitimate and the child of both of them. It is not difficult to imagine the complications which might arise, were a secret of this kind to leak out, but no case has yet been brought to court to raise the question of the legitimacy, and rights in respect of inheritance, of a child born of A.I.D.

Different views are held on the morality of A.I.D. To many the idea of it is distasteful on account of the conspiracy of silence involved, the questionable right of the child to inherit, and the mentality of the donor. Further, A.I.D. seems to some to approximate too closely to adultery. But the mother is the physical mother of her child which is biologically half hers, an argument which appeals to many liberal minds, and the husband has had the responsibility of providing for a pregnant wife and then for her new-born baby. She, too, conceived the child without sexual pleasure, while many women want sexual pleasure without children—an argument which can be adduced against any puritanical moralist.

The extent of the practice of A.I.D. cannot be ascertained. The conspiracy of silence is too close all round. But it seems reasonable to suppose that, although it has attracted little attention in spite of its now wide application in stock raising, there are now many genuine mothers today who would otherwise have been forced to adopt someone else's child.*

Compulsory restraint

Individual liberty has to be restricted in the interests of the health of society in many spheres, in that of drugs and driving, in that of the termination of pregnancy, in that of the sale and distribution of milk, food, and drink. Sometimes it has to be restricted altogether. Smallpox is so dangerous that under the law a case is removed compulsorily to hospital; indeed that of any notifiable fever, if the patient cannot be safely nursed at home. A criminal is put in prison, partly as a deterrent to others, partly as a deterrent to himself, partly in the usually vain hope of reforming his character, and also to render it impossible for him to do it again as long as he is held. Similarly a man living in an unreal world, a psychotic—hitherto called a lunatic—can be forcibly detained against his will if, as the result of his mental state, his actions are dangerous either to himself or others.

The existing attitude to, and the way of handling insanity, or rather mental ill-health—for that is what it is now called—is very recent. Until well into the nineteenth century, the concept of the lunatic as a man possessed lingered on, even if unspoken. Or at any rate he was regarded as alienated from his normal self —to use a word current at that time—and in need of segregation from society. An attitude of amused contempt persisted. So people who should not have been locked up, were locked up, or

* A.I.H. and A.I.D. may now, it seems, soon be possible the reverse way round in the sense that, if a woman is infertile by a fertile husband, an ovum could be obtained by ovarian puncture, either from her or from another woman, and then fertilized in a suitable medium in a test tube by her husband's semen. There it will develop as far as the blastula stage. Beyond this point embedding in the mucous membrane of a uterus, duly prepared to receive it, and placenta formation are both essential. It should be possible, however, to get a woman's uterus ready for implantation by the administration of progesterone, and implant the blastula in it mechanically, and then there is no theoretical reason why the embryo should not continue to develop normally, birth following when progesterone is withdrawn at full term. But between conception *in vitro* and the 'test tube baby' there is still a vast gap, and it is difficult to see how this will be bridged.

were kept locked up long after they had recovered. Indeed, not until 1890, common law having proved inadequate both to protect the mentally ill and to protect the public, was the Lunacy and Mental Treatment Act passed. This established asylums under a Board of Control, and by various provisions endeavoured to protect the public against danger, and the individual against wrongful detention.

In 1947 the Health Service took over these asylums, which changed their name to hospitals, and the Mental Health Act of 1959 brought both their administration and statute law in these matters into line with the new concept of mental disorder. Approbrious terms such as lunacy, insanity, asylums, were abrogated. The distinction between mental and physical illness lapsed. A reception order for detention replaced certification, and mental ill-health for judicial purposes was divided into four categories: the mentally ill, which included the functional and organic psychoses; the severely sub-normal, i.e. those who had never developed sufficiently in mind to be able to look after their bodies (formerly called mentally deficient); the sub-normal (formerly called feeble minded); and the psychopathic, i.e. the wrong-minded and socially irresponsible whether or not they were mentally sub-normal in addition. Further, compulsory detention, the 'certification' of former days, was taken out of the hands of the judiciary, in whose hands it used in part to rest, and handed over entirely to the medical profession. Two doctors can now sign a reception order for the compulsory detention of a person. But one must be his own general pracittioner and the other a mental specialist.

As the result of modern methods of treatment and this recent legislation, compulsory detention is now much less common than it used to be. The sub-normal and psychopathic, under the law as it now stands, cannot be detained against their will, if over the age of twenty-one. So in these days the risk of wrongful detention is small. Rather, the risk has shifted on to the other foot. It is sometimes too difficult now to get a reception order for a person on grounds of danger to himself or other people. Patients are also sometimes sent home prematurely, and too much responsibility imposed in consequence on those who remain under an obligation to look after them.

The problem of responsibility often arises. Is a certain person in a fit mental state to continue a responsible job? Is he fit to marry? Is he fit to make a will, or was he in his right mind when he made one? Is he fit to be a trustee of money or a guardian of a child? Doctors are often called upon to express opinion on these matters both in private practice and in courts of law. The question of criminal responsibility also arises. For the law accepts the view that a man is free within limits to choose between courses of action. On the other hand, it recognizes that the mind developed on the body is profoundly influenced by disease of it, and that at a certain point the power to choose lapses. Further, it realizes that a man can act on a pathological impulse of the moment, in epilepsy, for instance, or as the result of a fixed delusion which dominates his mind.

According to the McNaghten rules, which still hold in English courts, a man is liable for an unlawful act unless, either he did not know what he was doing at the time or, if he did know that, he did not know that what he was doing was wrong in the eyes of ordinary people. He might have been deluded, for example, and have believed that killing someone was necessary in the interests of humanity, but still know that he was acting contrary to law. So the rules go on to state that if, in spite of this belief, he knew that he was acting contrary to the law, he is criminally liable. Further, in order for insanity to be pleaded in his defence, his defect must be one of his *reason* due to a disease of his *mind*, although the law admits that this may be secondary to disease of his body. A special law relates to acts committed under the influence of drink.

These rules, as they stand, leave emotion out of account, and are an over-simplification of our concept of mind, which, of course, works as a whole. Intellect affects emotional feeling. Emotional feeling distorts intellect. In a psychotic depression a woman may murder her child, although she knew that this was morally wrong; and equally well what the consequences of her act would be. Further, the law talks about disease as if it was capable of definition, and of the mind as if it existed independently of the body, reflecting the fundamentally different approach to these matters of lawyers and doctors. The former want cut and dried answers to specific questions; it is convenient for the law to have the mind working in compartments. But the latter can seldom give them, and know that the mind works as a whole. One part of it cannot be affected without affecting the other. The classifications which man imposes on nature help his understanding of it but must not be pushed too far.

Ten years ago criminal law was amended in order to bring it more into line with modern concepts. In common law gross provocation has always led to a charge of murder being reduced to manslaughter. Under the Homicide Act of 1957 a plea of 'diminished responsibility' now reduces murder to manslaughter, 'if the accused was suffering from such abnormality of the mind as to substantially impair his sense of responsibility'. This allows disorder of emotional control to be pleaded in the defence of a man who has committed murder.

CHAPTER IX

PATIENT, DOCTOR, STATE

Preventive medicine—Health Service—Not feeling well—
Clinical diagnosis—Laboratory diagnosis—Therapeutics—
Transplant surgery—Psychiatric treatment—Meeting the
cost—Teaching and research.

The ordinary man looks to the State to protect him from risk
within reason and to the doctor, when he is ill and becomes a
patient, to get him well. The doctor looks to the patient to provide his livelihood, directly or through the State, and to the
State, under which he is registered and entrusted with certain
duties, to create the environment in which he can practise
efficiently. The State, primarily interested in maintaining the
labour force of the nation, and seeking a high standard of health
at low cost, looks to the ordinary man to play the game by the
services which it provides, and to the doctor to maintain them at
minimum cost. In some matters the interests of all three parties
coincide. In others they conflict. These three, patient, doctor
and society incorporated into the State, stand together in tri-
angular relationship.

Preventive medicine

The intervention of the State in matters relating to health is
really very recent. Even in this country it started little more than
a century ago, precipitated by the revolution which transformed
England from an agricultural community into an industrial
society and by the rapid increase of population which went with
it. The Factory Act of 1802, which controlled the hours of work
of women and children, marked the beginning of the movement
that, with the awakening of the social conscience, the zeal of the
reformers, the philosophy of Bentham and the Evangelical re-
vival, rapidly gathered momentum as the century advanced.

Child labour was made illegal; the hours of work in factories controlled. Reform of the Poor Law followed. Acts of Parliament ensured the main drainage and controlled the water supply of cities. Medical Officers of Health were started. Public houses were licensed and their hours of opening restricted. The inspection of ships and quarantine regulations were enforced; vaccination rendered readily available; the notification of diseases compelled; safety precautions laid down for factories and mines; the sale of poisons controlled; unemployment benefit and old age pensions instituted. And so on and so on, until in 1919 health matters were taken out of the hands of the Privy Council and handed over to a Department of State specifically responsible for them, and entrusted at its inception with the urgent problem of slum clearance and housing, both so important in the maintenance of health. Indeed, by the end of the First World War, during which the importance of manpower and a high standard of national health had been so clearly demonstrated, the principle had been conceded that the prevention of disease by the control of environment was a responsibility of government, and that a certain proportion of the national income must in future be devoted to it.

Since then, too, the social services have come into being. The general practitioner no longer works unaided in the prevention or treatment of disease. He now has all the services maintained by the local authority at his disposal. There are birth control clinics and family planning centres—married couples can even get expert genetic advice—innoculation, infant welfare and child guidance clinics, to which he can refer his patients, and the school medical and dental services with which he works in close co-operation. He can call in the district nurse when circumstances demand it. The midwife helps him to bring the infant into the world; the maternity nurse looks after the new baby. The health visitor takes over when she leaves, and working in conjunction with him sees that the services provided by central and local authorities are used to the best advantage of each family in the interests of their physical health.

Education in relation to health is more difficult. Many of the ills of modern society and much ill-health—obesity, coronary disease, bronchitis, for instance—can be attributed directly or indirectly to failure in the art of living. Health and educational authorities are, however, beginning to co-operate in an effort to fill this gap in education. Youth organizations, voluntary and State-aided, are endeavouring to cope with the problems created by broken homes, too much money, too little to do, and the related problems of drugs and psychopathic behaviour in the teenage group. Social psychiatric workers have been appointed in some districts, and co-operate with the probation officers appointed by the Home Office. Marriage guidance clinics have come into being in some places, but marriage guidance, although clearly important, is not yet recognized by local authorities as a branch of preventive medicine. The difficulty is to assess the return on money spent on health education, and it can be spent in so many directions. But it can be argued that money so spent would earn a bigger invisible dividend than the tangible but sometimes problematical benefits derived from some modern medicine and surgery.

Health Service

The intervention of the State in the treatment of disease is more recent still. Until half a century ago the poor, with the exception of paupers in the infirmaries, were entirely dependent on hospitals which had been founded by charity and were maintained by voluntary contribution. Not until 1912, did the National Insurance Act entitle every employed person with an income below a certain figure to free domiciliary treatment, financed out of contributions by the insured person and his employer, the balance of the cost being provided by the State. Not until 1929, did a Local Government Act transfer the Poor Law infirmaries to the local authorities, and enable men and women to be treated at them even if they were not destitute. And most countries now have some arrangement that provides free domiciliary and hospital treatment for those unable to pay for it themselves.

This country has gone further. In 1948 the National Health Act provided free domiciliary and hospital treatment for everyone, irrespective of income, and also brought all the hospitals, voluntary and rate-dependent, under the financial control of the State, the income for the Health Service to be derived in part from the contributions of employed persons, in part from the compulsory contributions of their employers, and in part, like housing, education and defence, out of the national income from direct and indirect taxation. Charity no longer plays a part in the treatment of the sick.

The doctor's position *vis-à-vis* his patient has therefore changed materially. He now derives his income, not only from his patients, but also from their employers and the State. So today the two latter can claim a share of his allegiance, and it is now as much his duty to protect them from exploitation by his patients, as it used to be to protect his patients from exploitation by them. In fact the general practitioner is now often in a position in which he must arbitrate between their interests, although his inclination must always be to take his patient's side. That is the tradition of his profession. But the hospital doctor, to whom the general practitioner refers a case, is likely to incline in the opposite direction. His inclination is to protect the State by saving the payment of sickness benefit, for example, or protect society by stopping a man driving who is not safe to drive. He has no particular allegiance to the patients sent to see him. They have not chosen him. Rather, the hospital which he serves, and through which he draws his salary, has done that, and it is maintained by the State.

Not feeling well

The average man believes himself to be in health when he feels subjectively and looks objectively, as he thinks that he should feel and look, indeed, as he would maintain that he ought and has the right to feel and look. Most men are satisfied if they feel and look today just as they did yesterday, and felt and looked yesterday just as they did the day before.

When, however, a man wakes up, and for no accountable reason does not feel his normal self, or during the day suddenly gets a sudden pain somewhere, for instance, or discovers something odd about his body, a combination of fear and common-sense combine to tell him that he would be wise to seek advice. When lesser symptoms start slowly, this decision may be more difficult. But in general it is one which a man can only take himself, and in most cases turns on the result of a conflict in his mind, against a background of half-knowledge, between fear, on the one hand, and wishful thinking on the other.

This difficulty is inherent in medicine, and there is no doubt as to the wisdom of routine examination in childhood. This detects early dental, eye and ear disease, and conserves teeth, hearing and vision. Routine radiography of the chest is also worthwhile in adolescence. But in later life the fear engendered by over concentration on health is balanced against the problematic gain of routine 'check-ups'. Clinical examination usually fails to reveal organic disease in the pre-symptomatic stage. Expensive and often uncomfortable laboratory or X-ray investigations are required for that, and these are out of the question as a routine. There are, of course, exceptions to this statement, notably routine examination in the early diagnosis of carcinoma of the breast and cervix, and patients who want an annual checkup are allowed to have it. But in general the health of the greatest number, in so far as this can be estimated, is achieved by encouraging a more robust attitude to life than that which generally prevails at present.

Three courses are open to a man who feels that he must seek advice. He can see the doctor with whom he is registered in the Health Service. This may mean waiting in a crowded surgery. So, if he can afford it, he may decide to see him as a private patient, in which case, having bought his time, he feels that he will get all the attention he requires. Thirdly, he can consult an exponent of one of those methods of treatment which are not recognized by the Health Service which has nailed its flag to the mast of orthodox medicine based on the inductive method of reasoning from organized observation and experiment.

Faith-healing is the most ancient, and ante-dates the dawn of history. And it often works. Symptoms, as we have seen, are often due to fear, and faith often casts out fear more readily than logic, the faith-healer often proving far more successful with functional disorders than the psychotherapist or doctor. Further, many of any doctor's successes are due to faith in him, or in what he gives or does, rather than to the actual consequences of anything he gave or did. Whether faith can cure organic disease is a difficult question, but some diseases regarded as organic are in part psychogenic, and there is little theoretical reason why it should not in these, provided that they have not gone too far. Certainly there is no theoretical reason why it should not stop them starting. Whether faith can lead to intervention of the divine, and cure any organic disease, remains a question of belief. Miracles have been claimed, particularly within the Roman Catholic Church, but the facts never seem quite convincing, and the original diagnosis is often to some extent in doubt. Christian Science denies the existence of evil. This is running away from reality, and the child of Christian Science parents, who refuse to call in a doctor, lives exposed to risk.

Homoeopathy was founded in the eighteenth century by Hahnemann, who had come to the conclusion that drugs tend to produce in health the same symptoms as they relieve in disease, the best drug to use, always being that which produces the same symptoms as those under treatment. This principle, rather than the minute dose, is the basis of homoeopathic belief, a faith to which the vast majority of doctors, with a scientific training behind them, cannot subscribe. A few manage to believe in it, although they seldom hesitate to employ orthodox methods as well. There are in fact medically qualified homoeopathists and homoeopathic hospitals. For homoeopathy appeals to those, and there are many of them, who react instinctively against scientific medicine, and prefer something with an element of mystery about it. Many homoeopathic doctors, too, are unconscious psychotherapists. They engage mainly in private practice, listen patiently, and give their patients plenty of time. This is often half the therapeutic battle, although the busy life of an ordinary G.P. does not always permit it.

Osteopathy was founded by Andrew Taylor Still in 1874 as a reaction against drugs. All disease, he held, was due to anatomical peculiarities, particularly of the hip and spinal column, leading to pressure on soft parts, and could be cured by manipulation. Osteopathy has, however, shifted its ground since Still's day. X-rays failed to reveal any bony lesions, and post-mortem examination did not show anything either. The modern osteopathic concept is functional rather than organic. The lesion is a 'strained joint', and on this theory osteopathy has built a pathology of disease which is entirely incompatible with orthodox concepts. Some osteopaths remain true to the pure faith of Still's gospel. All diseases are predisposed to, if not actually caused by, osteopathic lesions, but most now admit that the body is not entirely self-sufficient in respect of curing itself aided by osteopathic methods, and that modern surgical techniques are also sometimes necessary. Many successful osteopaths are medically qualified.

Manipulation is the basic technique of osteopathy, and many people, dissatisfied with orthodox medicine, resort to osteopaths. The wiser among the latter know their limitations. They refuse some cases. But anyone who consults an unorthodox practitioner in the first instance runs some risk. On the other hand, osteopaths often succeed after doctors fail. Some of these cures are due to a patient's faith in his osteopath. Others are due to unconscious suggestion on his part, and, like homoeopaths, many osteopaths are natural psychotherapists. Like them too, they are in private practice, and can give their patients plenty of time. Osteopathy 'on the State' would be much less successful than osteopathy in private practice. Osteopaths, however, not only possess faith in their methods, but also empirical knowledge and technical skill in manipulation which the average doctor does not, and the trained orthopaedic surgeon may not, possess. But his patient's faith is essential to his success, and the reason why doctors cannot appreciate the minutiae of osteopathic technique is largely due to the fact that these do not really matter.

All unorthodox practitioners can afford to take risks which the ordinary doctor cannot. For the latter are always fair game, and many people derive satisfaction out of becoming 'one up' on the medical profession. If the osteopath fails, the patient keeps his mouth shut. But if his doctor proves unsuccessful, he tells all his friends, and then seeks unorthodox advice, the success of which often coincides with the natural tendency of many conditions to remit with the passage of time.

Clinical diagnosis

Diagnosis is of necessity clinical in the first instance. For it depends on what the patient tells his doctor, and on what he finds on examining him by means of his unaided senses. And it is often much more difficult than might have been supposed. Few diseases present symptoms of which they have a monopoly and by which they can be recognized at sight.

As soon as a patient starts to talk, indeed even before that, particularly if he looks ill or in some way odd, a doctor's mind starts working. He listens to what he has to say but is soon prompted into asking him questions. If he complains of pain, he often concentrates more on when, rather than on where it is felt or on what it is like. For pain is difficult to locate and hard to describe, and *when* is often a better guide to its origin than *where* it is felt. Pain on breathing must originate in the lungs or in the muscles which move them; on exertion, in the heart; after meals, in the stomach or duodenum; related to bowel action, in the colon. Steady pain unrelated to functional demand, such as eating and exertion, may originate in an organ which is always in action like the liver and pancreas. Pain which is always with a person may also be psychogenic, turned on to serve some selfish purpose.

Proceeding in this way, a doctor soon has his patient sized up, and may come to the conclusion that his symptoms are constitutional. He has been over-taxing his digestion or powers of physical endurance. Alternatively, if his symptoms bear a relation to his emotional life, they may be psychogenic. More often their recent onset and relation to demand on function raise the probability of their organic origin in which case, as his patient talks, the doctor's mind starts working on two lines simultaneously. First, what do these symptoms, things of which his patient complains, and these signs, things he finds on examining him, mean in terms of the machinery of his body gone wrong? Secondly, what has put it wrong?

The same symptoms may be due to many disorders of function: shortness of breath, for example, to failure of any member of the triad responsible for getting oxygen to and carbon dioxide back from the tissues, and therefore to failure of the heart, lungs or blood. Jaundice, which people tend to think of as a disease, may be due to direct action on the liver, to obstruction of the bile duct (which may in turn be due to several causes), or to over-rapid destruction of the blood leading to excessive production of bile pigment. The same disorder of function may also be due to many actions on, and reactions by the body (i.e. to many different pathological processes). Loss of voice, which most people think of as laryngitis, may be adopted subconsciously to shirk work.

But it is usually due to virus, and occasionally to tuberculous or syphilitic, infection. During the First World War it was often due to mustard gas. Sometimes it turns out to be due to cancer. But it may be traumatic, merely the result of shouting at a football match!

When his patient complains of symptoms of a mental kind, a doctor adopts the same system of thinking. First, the nature of his mental state is assessed. He may be confused or have lost his memory. He may have hallucinations, seeing things that are not there, or be deluded, that is to say, in a state of false belief. He may be anxious, restless, excited, agitated, depressed. He may be withdrawn from the world, or merely appear so because his personality is inadequate. Then the most likely cause of it is thought out. Anxiety points to neurosis; intellectual defect to organic disease. Depression often proves to be due to something about which his patient is not prepared to talk. But it may prove to be endogenous. Excitement is usually psychotic. But it may be due to drugs or even to cerebral syphilis. If his patient is withdrawn from the world, and the doctor has difficulty in making contact with him, he suspects schizophrenic breakdown.

At least that, in so far as it can be described, is the way a doctor works when someone first comes to consult him, and clearly he is to a large extent dependent on his patient's good faith, memory and power of description. Few deliberately tell lies, but some exaggerate their symptoms, while others, having screwed up their courage, play them down in fear that they may prove to be of serious significance. But it is usually possible for him to make up his mind with a reasonable degree of confidence whether his patient is constitutionally weak, neurotic (his well-being at the mercy of his subsconscious), in a mental state, or suffering from organic disease. Further, he can usually make up his mind in the latter case as to the way in which the machinery of his patient's body has gone wrong; whether his heart is failing, for example, or his thyroid over-acting. The cause of it is more difficult to assess, although that is sometimes clear, as in symptoms dating from birth, from an accident, or following exposure to infection. Further, pathological processes tend to affect the body at different ages, and to affect one sex more often than the other. Many also tend to produce characteristic combinations of alteration of structure and disturbance of function. They have habits by which they can be recognized at sight.

Clinical diagnosis, like many other branches of human activity, obeys the law of diminishing returns. By taking reasonable care a doctor can spot, say, 75 per cent of cases of some potentially dangerous disease among patients coming to consult him; and another 20 per cent by being scrupulously careful. The remaining 5 per cent, it must be admitted, are often not recognized at a first visit. Occasional mistakes are in fact inevitable. For although a general practitioner knows that a man or woman beginning to suffer from something serious is bound to turn up every now and again in his surgery, he is always pressed for time, another patient always treading on the tail of his last one, impatient to be seen. Further, it is not those who are organically ill that take up most of it. They are often easy in the sense that it is clear what is the matter with them, and often also clear what should be done about them. It is the neurotic, and those wanting to be ill, who take up most of it, and organic disease may lurk behind the scenes even in them. It is when a neurotic starts to develop organic disease that a serious mistake is most likely to be made.

Laboratory diagnosis

The general practitioner, in the front line of medicine in the sense that most illness comes his way in the first instance, always makes some sort of diagnosis, and then estimates his chances of being right, although he often only does the latter unconsciously. For on this depends what he does about his patient next.

In most cases he can rely on his often quick assessment of a mental or physical state, based on what his patient tells him and on what he finds on examining him, as a reasonable basis for action. Many conditions are obvious at sight. Or anyhow not much thinking is required. And, of course, until recently, even in a difficult case, this was all a doctor had to go on. But now, as the result of the application of the techniques of scientific research to clinical problems, it is usually possible to confirm, extend or disprove a clinical diagnosis by X-rays, blood tests, biopsies, microscopic examination, chemical analyses, electrical recordings and other methods, collectively known as investigations, or exclude some fear haunting the back of a doctor's mind. For doctors suffer from fear, like their patients, fear easily communicated to them; the fear of making a mistake, particularly that of attributing symptoms to a functional disorder when they are really due to organic disease. A doctor may be afraid, too, of making the mistake the other way round; of attributing symptoms to organic disease when they are really nervous in origin. The first is far and away the graver mistake. Treatment may be delayed in consequence, the opportunity to save a life actually let slip.

A general practitioner always sticks to, and acts on, his clinical diagnosis, and starts treating his patient accordingly, if he feels he can with reasonable safety. For investigations take time and cost money. Commonsense dictates that they must be used with reasonable discretion and with due regard to economy. Every patient cannot have every test or X-ray which might prove relevant to his condition. A doctor can never play for absolute safety. Too much anxiety would be caused in the minds of too many, and in most cases a clinical diagnosis is a sufficient basis for action. When he feels less confident, but decides that he has time in hand, he may give the disease he suspects time to declare itself. In many of these cases symptoms have remitted by the time his patient comes back to see him. Procrastination has spared expense, and saved unnecessary discomfort. Sometimes a doctor's fear does of course prove to have been justified. But, if a second visit is not delayed too long, serious harm is seldom done.

In other cases the diagnosis on clinical grounds is not clear, nor clear even on a second visit. Some point must be settled; some serious possibility excluded. But, as would be expected, there are border-line cases, and the decision as to whether to have this or that test done, or this or that X-ray taken, and making up his mind as to whether he ought to send his patient to hospital for investigation, may be very difficult. There is no rule of thumb guide to decisions of this kind. They are human judgments. Just as a man must make up his own mind whether it is really necessary to seek medical advice, so a doctor must make up his own mind as to whether it is really necessary to have his patient investigated.

Admission to hospital for investigation means a trying time

for a patient. He has to wait to come in. Then he waits from day to day wondering what is to be done next, and when a final verdict will be pronounced. Will his worst fears, or perhaps the fear that he has sensed in his doctor's mind, be realized? So, during this period, his morale must be maintained. The diagnosis in these circumstances demands an assessment of his mental state in relation to his illness. This dictates how he is handled.

Therapeutics

In theory, diagnosis should precede treatment. How can a doctor prescribe for his patient's needs until he knows what is the matter with him? But this statement only applies to the pathological process behind the scenes, not to the disorder of function resulting from it which may dominate the situation. Consciousness may have suddenly lapsed, because breathing or the heart has stopped, and then whichever it is must be got going again irrespective of its cause. That can be found out later. Or a man may be so anaemic that he must be transfused merely to keep him alive. Further, functional disorders such as a cough, pain, vomiting and diarrhoea must be controlled, pending the diagnosis of their cause.

Pain is the commonest symptom and, being an event in consciousness, is to some extent under voluntary control. It is reduced by self-discipline and aggravated by lack of emotional control, and can sometimes be abolished by hypnosis. A tooth can be extracted in 25 per cent of people under hypnosis. But it is an uncertain method. In the vast majority of cases pain is more satisfactorily controlled by means of drugs.

In malnutrition, dehydration, and vitamin deficiency, treatment presents no particular difficulties. The important thing is to start it. Rickets untreated for too long leads to irreversible skeletal deformity, and the intestinal tracts of many of the victims rescued from Belsen at the end of the war had grown so intolerant of food that they died, it can almost be said, as the result of being fed.

In severe injury arterial bleeding is stopped first, then the airway cleared, and then shock and its associated fall of blood pressure countered by giving blood, plasma, or saline. Amputation or excision of a wound may be necessary when sufficient recovery from shock has rendered it safe, and plastic surgery and skin grafting may be necessary later.

In acute poisoning the offending substance must be eliminated. If it has been swallowed, an emetic is given. If it has been injected, or has already been absorbed, elimination is promoted through the kidneys by giving large quantities of water and, in barbiturate poisoning, by repeated lumbar puncture. If an antidote is known, it is given at once. The functional consequences of the poison are always countered. Barbiturates depress breathing, and respiration must be maintained. Strychnine tends to convulsions. These can be countered by drugs which depress the nervous system, or rendered impossible by curare which paralyses motor nerve endings.

In infection the inborn reactions to it are encouraged. Inflammation, the reaction to local infection, is stimulated by the application of heat. Fever, the reaction to general infection, is left to run its course. Infection is also sometimes treated surgically; an abscess opened, for example, or an acutely inflamed appendix or chronically inflamed tonsils excised. The treatment of acute infection also often depends on its nature. When, as in diphtheria and tetanus, it is associated with toxin production, the effects of that are countered by giving antitoxin. More often treatment is directed against the organisms themselves, either by giving a chemotherapeutic agent which kills them without harming the body—for example, one of the sulphonamides in streptococcal infection and isoniazid in tuberculosis; or an antibiotic produced by a fungus, for instance, penicillin in streptococcal infection and streptomycin in tuberculosis. But chemotherapy is not as simple as it often sounds. Many of these agents have unwanted side-effects, and it is difficult to know to which one the infecting organism will prove susceptible. Further, just as man develops resistance to infection, so organisms develop resistance to antibiotics. There is in fact the risk that the present indiscriminate use of the antibiotics will lead to pathogenic organisms becoming resistant to most of them. Some therefore think that some of our new ones should be kept in reserve against the day when organisms, which have developed immunity to the rest, start to cause disease which we shall otherwise find ourselves powerless to control.

Many diseases are not yet understood. We do not know their cause or, as it is probably more correct to say, we do not understand the many factors which have conspired to produce them. But some of them, at least, are amenable to treatment in the sense that the patient can be kept free, or nearly free, of symptoms, although it cannot be claimed that he has been restored to normal health.

Many congenital malformations can be repaired, some with almost complete success; cleft palate, for instance, restoring a normal quality to the voice, and hare lip, leaving a scar which is barely noticeable. Most of congenital malformation of the heart can also be satisfactorily repaired. Malformation of the nervous system due to failure of the spinal canal to close is less satisfactory to treat, and considerable loss of function is often left behind. But we can seldom remedy genetic defects of a functional kind. We cannot restore normal clotting to haemophilic blood, or give a mongol child a normal brain on which to develop its mind.

Many acquired diseases, although again we do not know their cause, can be treated. A potential cretin put on daily thyroid grows up an almost normal child, and when a woman develops myxoedema, she can be kept free of symptoms by the same method. Addison's disease, due to failure of the suprarenal cortex, can be successfully treated by giving cortisone, and although diabetes is not due to simple failure of pancreatic function, most cases can be kept in normal health by means of daily insulin. Diseases due to unexplained over-action of function can also often be successfully treated. Thyrotoxicosis, for instance, the symptoms of which are due to over-action of the thyroid, can be handled, either by reducing thyroxine secretion by removing part of the gland, or by giving drugs known to antagonize its action. Haemolytic anaemia can be relieved by removing the spleen, and over-production of red corpuscles in the marrow by irradiating the bones. Although we do not know what causes arterial constriction, increasing the resistance to the flow of blood and necessitating rise of blood pressure, we now possess drugs that reduce this constriction, and therefore lower it, prolonging the life of the arteries and conserving that of the heart and kidneys. The hypersensitivity diseases benefit from immuno-suppressive drugs.

When a disease is localized, and situated where it can be cut out without interfering with any vital function, this is done, if no other method of treatment is available. Part of the stomach is sometimes removed in gastric ulcer, and the whole colon in ulcerative colitis. Excision is also still the method of election in the treatment of malignant growth, provided it is diagnosed before it has given rise to secondaries elsewhere. But malignant cells are more sensitive than normal cells to ionizing radiation and, although the margin is small, X-rays, radium and other radio-active elements are now used alone in inoperable, or in conjunction with surgery, in operable cases. Operations for cancer are much less radical now than they were a short time ago, and surgery is not always necessary. The growth of carcinoma of the prostate and breast, two common forms of cancer, is slowed down by castration, while a similar although less satisfactory result can be achieved by physiological castration, that is to say, by giving female hormone to the male and male hormone to the female. Their rate of growth can be reduced still further by removing the suprarenals, or alternatively by removing the anterior lobe of the pituitary which drives the suprarenals into action.

Orthopaedic and plastic surgery, and mechanical and physical devices, compensate for many structural defects and many failures of function irrespective of their cause. An artificial leg compensates for a lost limb, and a diseased joint can be fixed in the optimum position, or a new one sometimes fashioned. Plastic and metal joints are now both used. In paralysis, a nerve can sometimes be transferred from some unimportant to some more important function. Braille enables the blind to read by touch. Sound can be amplified, enabling the deaf to hear. Spectacles correct errors of refraction, and take the place of the lens after that has been removed for cataract.

When the heart stops and breathing ceases, a man is no longer necessarily deemed dead. His lungs can be operated by the mouth to mouth method of artificial respiration (or mechanically through an intra-tracheal tube) and a sufficient circulation often maintained by external cardiac massage. Then his heart will sometimes start again naturally, or it can be restarted electrically as soon as the apparatus is available. But the higher centres are peculiarly sensitive to lack of oxygen, and resuscitation is sometimes only successful at the expense of permanent mental defect.

In cessation of cardiac action (asystole) due to drowning, electrocution, chemical poisoning, and the heart stopping during an operation, many lives have now been saved by this method. In the latter the stage is already sometimes set so as to permit internal cardiac massage, i.e. grasping the heart in the hand and squeezing it rhythmically, as opposed to applying pressure to the chest wall over it, pressure which, to effect its purpose, must be so strong that it sometimes fractures ribs. In other cases of asytole the cause lies in the heart itself. The bundle of tissue connecting the auricles with the ventricles suddenly fails to conduct the stimulus to contract from the former, where it is generated, to the latter. Then the ventricles can sometimes be started beating at their own rate of about thirty by electrical stimulation; or, if they cannot be restarted, or keep stopping, they can be kept beating by means of an artificial pace-maker and a battery grafted under the skin. More often the ventricles stop beating, not because impulses fail to reach them, but because one of the coronary arteries (which supply the heart with blood) has been suddenly blocked with the result that part of the heart muscle (the infarcted area) is suddenly deprived of oxygen. Even under these circumstances, however, if sufficient circulation can be maintained by external cardiac massage, the heart may start to beat again of its own accord, or it can sometimes be induced to do so by electrical stimulation, provided too much damage has not been done.*

In acute renal failure due to a cause from which a patient has a chance of recovery, acute nephritis, for instance, life can sometimes be saved by haemodialysis. In chronic renal failure due to congenital cystic disease, bilateral destruction by stone forma-

---

* In many cases of this latter type muscular activity has not ceased. Rather the ventricles have gone into fibrillation, a condition in which their constituent fibres, instead of contracting together, all contract irrespective of each other, the net result of which is lack of any effective beat. Normal beating can however often be restored by a strong electric shock applied through the chest. Cases of ventricular fibrillation in fact do better than those of cessation of ventricular activity because, while fibrillation is often due to a small, cessation of vetricular activity is usually due to a large infarct.

tion, and chronic nephritis, it can be prolonged by the same method. Two tubes giving access to an artery and a vein are fitted in an arm or leg, and joined together so that the blood flows freely through this so-called shunt. Then, twice a week for about twelve hours, the tubes are linked up to a dialyser which now clears the body of urea in much the same way as does the normal kidney. The apparatus is expensive, the capital cost per hospital patient about £500, and maintenance about £1,500 per annum. (Haemodialysis at home costs several times as much.) Artificial kidney units are therefore few and far between, and cases are selected from among those that might benefit, the question of worthwhileness entering into both the more generous provision of haemodialysis units and into the selection of cases. A patient must also be emotionally stable to stand up to it. Many, although both their liberty and their diet are seriously restricted, manage to lead a more or less normal life on it. Some work, and women can often look after their children. But complications, particularly virus hepatitis, are not uncommon, and in renal failure due to chronic nephritis it is only possible to prolong life by a few years. The artificial kidney is seldom the miracle that the public has sometimes been led to suppose, and it looks now as if its main use will prove to be to keep a patient with chronic renal failure alive, pending the transplantation into him of a donor's kidney.

Transplant surgery

For the latest method of prolonging life in the face of failure of a vital function is to cut that organ on which it depends out, and graft in another from a healthy man.

When a large area of the body has been denuded, skin is taken from some other part of it, or from some other person, and spread over the denuded area. The former continues to live. The latter provides a temporary dressing while the patient regenerates his own which grows in slowly from the edges of his wound. Much the same is true of bone. Autonomous grafts live on but tissue of any kind from a donor, other than from an identical twin, is always to some extent antigenic to the recipient, and is slowly destroyed or, as it is now often put, rejected. But recently it has been discovered that this property can be much reduced by the technique of 'freeze-drying'. Tissue so treated allows more time for regeneration, and permits far more complex repair operations than would otherwise be possible. This process also permits tissue to be stored outside the body for long periods without deteriorioration, and tissue banks are now maintained in most countries. These dole out skin, peritoneum, nerve and bone to surgeons when and as required.

There are four main blood groups, and the blood of a man in one group is antigenic to a man in another with the result that, if he is transfused with it, he proceeds to destroy it, or in modern popular terminology to reject it, leading to haemolytic jaundice (incompatible blood transfusion). A man can in fact only be transfused with blood in the same group as that to which his own belongs. But this is now common and safe practice. Cross typing is easy. There are willing donors, and although there are rare groups, blood can be stored outside the body for long periods, and that of the right group issued from a central blood bank when and as required. Further, there is nothing permanent about blood transfusion. We are all always destroying our own blood—the average life of a red blood corpuscle is of the order of a month—and so, as would be expected, the donor's blood, although of the same group as the recipient's, is slowly destroyed too, and replaced by blood of his own making.

Corneal transplantation, although more permanent, also presents few problems. The donor is dead, and a sufficient number of people direct in their wills that their cornea may be used for this purpose. Further, corneal tissue is so avascular that no serious rejection problem arises.

The kidney was the first whole organ to be transplanted, and kidney grafting is now considered a more satisfactory alternative to haemodialysis in incurable kidney disease. But it is a responsibility for a doctor to undertake to persuade a relative to surrender his spare kidney. Anyone might get disease in that one left behind. On the other hand, if a functional kidney is to be obtained from a dead body, it must be taken out within an hour or so of death, and a kidney cannot be kept alive outside the body. In spite of these difficulties practice is swinging away from the live donor in the direction of a kidney from a dead man.

Unless the donor is an identical twin of the recipient, his kidney is always antigenic to some extent to him, and the latter starts to react in such a way as to destroy it. Therefore he has to be kept on drugs which suppress these reactions. These are of three kinds: steroids, i.e. substances related chemically to the internal secretion of the suprarenal cortex, chemicals destroying lymphocytes (the non-granular white cells of the blood which produce antibodies when antigens get into us), and antilymphocytic serum which does the same thing in a rather different way. But, as these all inhibit the normal reactions of the body to infection, a patient on them must also be kept on antibiotics. Therefore, living on a transplanted kidney, particularly as both antibiotics and immuno-suppressive drugs may have unwanted side effects, is far from a normal life. Those who have received a kidney from an identical twin donor do best. There is no rejection reaction, and some have already lived ten years. Those who have received kidneys from near relatives do relatively well. Rejection reactions are less intense than in the case of unrelated donors, and survival up to seven years has been recorded already. When the donor was no blood relation, survival up to four years after the operation is the best recorded yet. But at present all recipients of kidneys, except those in which the donor was an identical twin, seem destined to die sooner or later of a combination of rejection and infection.

The transplantation of the heart is technically more difficult. Further, the recipient has to be kept alive while his own heart is removed, pending the transfer of the donor's; and this involves maintaining his circulation by means of a heart-lung machine. The problem of rejection is also difficult since, as a heart can only be obtained from another man who has just died, again there is little time for tissue typing. The selection of patients in whom the tremendous undertaking of cardiac transplantation is really worth attempting is also difficult. Congenital malformation which cannot be satisfactorily repaired, advanced rheumatic heart disease in young subjects, and the myopathies found in the coloured races, would seem suitable cases. The worthwhileness of it in coronary disease is problematical. For that is merely one manifestation of general arterial disease, and it is impossible to survey the whole body from that aspect with any approximation to accuracy. When is it really justifiable, either from the point of view of expense or from that what a patient must endure, to transplant a 'new' heart—no hearts are ever really new—into a man or woman who might fall seriously ill in some other way within a comparatively short time?

Both lungs have now been transplanted, alone and also in conjunction with the heart to which they belong, and, as would be expected, in view of the relatively simple nature of lung tissue, a membrane carrying blood vessels, the rejection problem is not great. This tends to be outweighed, however, by the fact that transplanted lungs, being open to the air, are liable to become infected soon after transplantation.

The liver has also been transplanted, the indications for it being chemical damage, chronic inflammation, and primary cancer, the latter a rare disease. Surgically the operation is more difficult than cardiac transplantation. For the liver is tucked away high up under the diaphragm, and linking up the blood vessels of the donor's liver with the recipient's circulation is tricky. On the other hand, the rejection problem is not so great as might have been expected in view of the complicated functions of liver cells. In some animals, liver can be transplanted from one to another without any signs of rejection.

Recently a larynx, which contains the vocal cords, has been transplanted into a man, whose own larynx had been removed for cancer, and the cut ends of the nerves which operated his larynx sutured to the cut ends of the nerves in the donor's. But only time will show whether the recipient's laryngeal nerves, growing down from where they were divided and following the path of the degenerating nerves in the donor's larynx to which they have been sutured, will link up satisfactorily with the muscle fibres which operated the donor's vocal cords, and enable the recipient to speak aloud again.

Organ transplantation, appealing to the morbid interest of the public, is of commercial news value, and has engendered different emotions. Some see it as another triumph, another step towards the prolongation of life, a further advance in the direction of a brave new world of super minds based on patched-up bodies. Others react instinctively against it. Just as they believe in the value of the integrity of the mind, so they believe in that of the body, and view the idea of living on by means of organs belonging to other people with distaste.

The former fail to realize that, although the transplantation of the kidney has already found its place in medicine, it is not the real solution to the problem of kidney disease, while transplantation of the heart, even when that of rejection has been solved and the technique of it perfected, is likely to remain, for reasons already given, a rarely worthwhile operation. The latter must remember that the ethics of transplantation was conceded when blood transfusion was accepted, and how many of them would object to that, or hesitate to give their own blood when the life of a near relative was at stake, or refuse to accept a corneal graft when they themselves were going blind? Organ transplantation in fact does not raise, as many seem to think, new ethical problems, provided, of course, that the donor of a heart or liver is dead, and every effort was made to keep him alive, unless in *his* interest striving to do so had ceased to be worth while. Rather, what transplant surgery does do, indeed, has done already, is to bring to a head a problem which has been steadily growing more difficult with recent advances in medical science, namely, the worthwhileness in terms of the kind of life it prolongs, and the wisdom of spending large sums of money on the prolonging of one life when that money might be used to prevent disease in or help the lives of many others.*

There is seldom any doubt when a man dies. In progressive malnutrition, in increasing dehydration, in uncontrolled infection, in gradual heart and renal failure, in the last stages of malignant disease, there comes a moment when, as the coordination of function finally breaks down, respiration and circulation, being interrelated, fail more or less together. Heartbeat and breathing now cease simultaneously, and the oxygen supply to the tissues fails. This is the generally accepted moment of death.

* The transplantation of the brain would raise a new ethical issue. For the brain is the organ of the mind developed during life, and in it personality is vested. Transplantation of the brain would not be to keep the recipient's body alive. Rather, it would be keeping the donor's personality alive in someone else's body. But we need not bother about this yet. It does not lie in the foreseeable future. Not only would the technical difficulties be enormous, but it is impossible to see at present how for physiological reasons the donor's brain could be linked up with the recipient's body.

Consciousness, if the patient was still conscious, lapses. His pupils dilate, his jaw drops, his muscles go flaccid. Disintegration, first of function and then of structure, as oxygen supply fails generally, now sets in, but sets in more rapidly in the brain than in any other organ, nervous tissue being more oxygen dependent than any other. The doctor now knows from experience that his patient is dead in the sense that he knows that it is useless to attempt to resuscitate him, that is to say, to try to get heart and respiration restarted, as he would in a case of sudden *primary* cessation of cardiac action (p. 68). The whole man is dead, although, if action is taken sufficiently quickly, certain tissues, notably cornea, bone and skin, and even whole organs, heart, kidney, liver, can be kept alive for grafting into other patients. Death is, in fact, a clinical diagnosis, and the only cases in which any doubt arises are those of prolonged unconsciousness in which the life of the body is being maintained by mechanical ventilation of the lungs after the brain, on which the mind depends, has ceased to function. Whether a man in this condition can, after sufficient time has been allowed for recovery, be regarded as dead, awaits a decision of the courts or an Act of Parliament. When all cerebral activity has ceased, as judged by permanent absence of all waves on the electro-encaphalogram, he should certainly be regarded as dead. Death must be defined, in future, in terms of the mind developed on the body, rather than in terms of the body which maintains the mind.

Anyone is free to accept any organ or tissue of another person, provided it is legally given. Anyone is also free during his life to give away one of his organs or some of his tissue, provided that the operation to obtain it, and the operation to transplant it, can both be justified legally by the common law doctrine of necessity. Legal problems only arise when a man is dead. By the Anatomy Act of 1832, a man can direct that his body be examined after his death, although relatives can effectively object. By the Corneal Grafting Act of 1952, he can request that his eyes should be used for this purpose. But a dead body does not constitute property in law, and a man cannot dispose of his by will. Nor can his next-of-kin give away his organs when he is unconscious, even if there seems no hope of his recovery. When he is dead, however, under the Human Tissue Act of 1961 'the person lawfully in possession of the body of a deceased person may authorize the removal of any part of it for the said purpose if, having made such reasonable enquiries as may be practicable, he has no reason to believe that the deceased person had expressed any objection or that his surviving spouse or any surviving relative object to the body being so dealt with.'

The most suitable donors for organ transplantation are young people who have died as the result of physical injury. Their organs are both healthy and young. But cases of this kind are relatively few and far between, and one may not be available just when required. Indeed, at present enough kidneys for transplantation into all the patients with chronic renal failure whose lives might thereby be prolonged are not yet available. This is partly due to public prejudice against it and partly due to the fact that permission must be obtained to use a dead person's kidney for this purpose, and this takes time to get. (Some maintain that the law should be altered so as to allow it, if no objection is known to exist.) But the main difficulty arises out of the fact that functional tissue, such as kidney, liver and heart muscle, deteriorates much more rapidly after being taken out of the body than structural tissue, such as skin membrane and bone. So, although a potential kidney recipient can be kept waiting on haemodialysis, the donor's kidney must be grafted into him as quickly as possible after it has been taken out of the donor's body. The donor must therefore be in or have died in the same hospital as the recipient. Organ banks, comparable to tissue banks, do not yet exist. But functional deterioration, it has recently been discovered, can be delayed for some days by rapid freezing and also by certain chemical agents. This discovery, it is hoped, will in due course allow both time for tissue typing, as this is gradually perfected, and also time for a donor's organ to be flown from the hospital in which he died to the hospital in which it is to be grafted into a recipient.

Psychiatric treatment

Symptoms of a mental kind sometimes compel the segregation of patients from society. This, and the existence of the psychiatrist, who figures large in modern life, have conspired to create the impression that there must be some fundamental difference between psychiatric and other forms of medical treatment. But few mental states are treated by psychological methods alone. For the mind can be influenced through the brain as well as through the ordinary channels of communication between man and man. In practice these two methods—the physical, usually empirical, and the psychological, essentially rational—are usually combined.

The treatment of mental states due to organic disease (the organic psychoses) turns on the treatment of it, when a method of treating it exists, while the patient is controlled by means of drugs, or, if he is a danger either to himself or others, kept under restraint. Dementia, due to vitamin deficiency, for example, responds to vitamin B; mania, due to cerebral syphilis, to anti-syphilitic treatment.

The treatment of mental states in which some constitutional peculiarity predisposes the mind to succumb, endogenous depression, schizophrenia, etc. (the functional psychoses), on the other hand, remains empirical. Repeated lowering of the blood sugar by injecting insulin was thought at one time, erroneously it now seems, to benefit schizophrenia. Then convulsions produced by means of drugs, and later by electrical stimulation of the cortex (in these days actual convulsions are suppressed by injection of curare), were found to cut short endogenous depression. A few years ago division of the fibres connecting the prefrontal lobes with the brain stem (leucotomy) was found to render delusions, obsessions and states of agitation less disturbing. Recently a number of drugs have been introduced. Some counter depression, others tranquillize the mind, and these have gone some way towards replacing leucotomy. Some of these methods of treatment have gradually fallen out of use. But all have had their day, and combined collectively to lead to that increasing interest in, and growing optimism as to the outcome of mental illness, which have culminated in the attitude to it now prevailing. Indeed, it is these empirical methods, rather than rational psychotherapy, combined with the gradual realization that psychotic manifestations in mental institutions *may* be due to the conditions under which their inmates are confined, which have largely emptied, humanized, and unlocked the doors of our one-time prison-like mental asylums.

Further, of recent years the concept of social psychiatry, both in the prevention and treatment of mental illness, has steadily gained ground. Many patients benefit from organization into selected groups in which they discuss their troubles with each other and with their doctors and nurses on equal terms. Every effort is also made to rehabilitate them in relation to the demands of social living, when they eventually return home, and to restore their respect in themselves by means of work and hobbies. Neurosis, it is also now realized, is mainly, and schizophrenia partly, due to environmental factors. (Every race and culture has its own peculiar mental disorders.) So the prevention of mental disease, and its treatment in the early stages, must clearly always lie, it is now seen, largely in the province of the general practitioner, social worker, probation officer, and organizations devoted to particular problems such as marriage guidance, helping alcoholics, and protecting those in states of depression from themselves. In this extended sense it clearly links up with character training in schools, in the services, and even in certain walks of adult life.

Psychotherapy is of use in mental states of psychogenic origin in so far as any dividing line can be drawn between neurosis and psychosis. Every doctor, particularly a general practitioner, practises it, often to a very large extent unconsciously. It is part of his attitude to his patients and of the atmosphere he intentionally creates. When deliberately applied, it involves gaining a patient's confidence and getting him to tell the truth, and so finding out his fears, worries and difficulties, and then, having got him to understand himself better, helping him to help himself to solve his problems or adapt himself more successfully to the life which he has to lead, which probably cannot be altered, and which often seems so futile. It depends on reason, explanation, and suggestion, the methods all adopt in their daily dealing with their fellow men, combined with sympathy and kindliness. In organic medicine, diagnosis precedes treatment. In psychological medicine, it is treatment. Talking about something, and not keeping it to himself any longer, often helps a person to make the best of his circumstances. Much, of course, depends on the relationship which a doctor can establish with his patient. This turns on his capacity for insight into the minds of others, and his ability to appreciate their troubles, gifts possessed in different degrees by different people the importance of which tends to be neglected in the early education of the doctor with its concentration on the scientific approach to the problems of medical practice.

With the advent of psychotherapy, hypnotism, which has been recognized now for nearly two hundred years and which was much used by the French neurologists in the nineteenth century as a method of curing hysterical symptoms, has largely dropped out of fashion. Hypnotic shows and the like have prejudiced many people, both doctors and laymen, against it. It is also too individual. Some people are easy, others more difficult to hypnotize, and doctors hesitate or lack the confidence to try. Further, although it gets rid of symptoms, it leaves the personality structure unchanged, and is symptomatic medicine only, making no attempt to get at the underlying pathology. Symptoms treated by hypnosis tend to recur, or the patient develops new ones, when the circumstances of his life demand that he must escape from something again. Either therefore he must be repeatedly hypnotized, with the result that he becomes dependent on his hypnotist, or it must be combined with some other form of treatment. Hypnosis is, however, sometimes useful as a way of getting started. It breaks down the barrier between doctor and patient. In loss of memory, too, it may be a way of arriving at the truth. For under it, also sometimes under light anaesthesia, a person may remember some emotional experience through which he has passed and which is continuing to disturb his conscious life, but he has actively forgotten. It is also sometimes used to calm an agitated, obsessed or anxious person, as an alternative to drugs, pending exact diagnosis and the organization of some other more satisfactory or elaborate form of treatment.

Psychoanalysis, which dates from Sigmund Freud and the turn of the last century, is the antithesis of hypnotism. For it endeavours to get down to rock bottom of a person's mind, and discover the cause of and ascertain the nature of the basic defect in his personality which is responsible for his symptoms. But, while hypnotism is quick, psychoanalysis is time-consuming, entailing long interviews at frequent intervals extending over months or even years. Further, while hypnotic power is a gift, psychoanalysis demands training and practice in certain techniques, the free association of ideas, the interpretation of dreams and others. The patient is encouraged to talk and recall early memories and experiences, sexual and otherwise, which the analyst tries to relate to his patient's psychic life, the theory being that if he sees for himself how his mind has developed as the result of his experience, and comes to understand the origin of his fears, prejudices and inhibitions, he will react to experience in the future better than he has reacted to it in the past. But few patients can afford either the time for it or the money to pay for it. Only for very few can psychoanalysis ever be provided by the State.

Psychoanalysis has shed a flood of light on the working of the mind, and in so doing has conspired with other methods to engender the recent more sympathetic attitude to mental illness. But as a method of treatment it is difficult, indeed almost impossible, to assess. Statistical comparison of its results are out of the question. Control experiments can never be performed. For on the basis of its own claim to success a patient reacts differently after it to the way in which he reacted before it. A dream cannot be interpreted a second time, or the same patient analysed twice over. Further, it is not without risk. The revelation of self to self can be too disturbing, and mud stirred up in the mind may fail to settle. Like any form of sympathetic psychotherapy it can help a patient to adapt himself to circumstances, but biological science and psychoanalytical practice have revealed that personality is built in far too firmly and deeply in the early years to be altered much by any psychological method at a later date. (Only religious conversion, some claim, succeeds in doing that.) There is little evidence, for instance, that the direction of psychosexual development can be altered. A homosexual can be helped, but seldom cured.

In general practice time is the main commodity in short supply. Faced with the problem of a neurotic patient a doctor must often choose between drugs, reassurance, and referring him to the psychological department of a hospital. Some neurotic people regain their emotional equilibrium unaided. Their lapse was a passing phase. Others resent a doctor probing too deeply into their emotional affairs. So he often tries drugs. But he does not want to make his patient drug-minded, and yet the last thing he wants to do is to send him for psychological treatment unnecessarily. Any patient referred to a psychologist is forced to concede that he is no longer able to manage his own mind, and is one down in his self-esteem in consequence. Half an hour of the doctor's own time may be more worthwhile than all the organized psychotherapy available.

Meeting the cost

The Health Service costs a great deal. Further, the cost of it is steadily increasing. In terms of real money it costs many times more now than it did at its inception twenty years ago.

A doctor in general practice spends the income of it every time he writes a prescription or orders an appliance for one of his Health Service patients. He is limited, of course, in what he can do to some extent. He can be hauled over the coals for excessive prescribing, and must render an account of the dangerous drugs he dispenses. Further, he is under an obligation not to prescribe the more expensive drugs when cheaper ones will serve, and to avoid proprietary preparations when comparable National Health Formulary ones are available. But the pressure of his patients' requests is always tending to force him into prescribing. It is difficult to refuse pleas for tonics and sleeping pills; always easiest, particularly when he is rushed or tired, to give the patient what he wants; always less time-consuming, and certainly less exacting in terms of mental effort, to be 'sloppy' in diagnosis, and evade responsibility by ordering investigations. Besides, he plays for safety in so doing. Often, too, a patient expects an X-ray, and it takes time to convince him that it is really unnecessary; always easier to send him to, and shelter behind, the hospital, rather than bother to make up his own mind in a difficult case. Further, he spends public money every time he certifies a man unfit for work in terms of sickness or unemployment benefit.

The hospital doctor is under no such discipline. He has all the resources of modern medicine at his disposal, but the authority who appointed him has no real control over his use of them. If a patient needs this or that, the expert says, it is impossible for a lay committee to gainsay it, and many doctors working in hospitals are innocently unaware of the cost of many of the tests, investigations and X-rays which they order freely. Further, although careful clinical diagnosis makes for economy in investigational medicine, in most hospitals the initial sorting of patients is left to junior staff with little experience. Large numbers of investigations are ordered quite unnecessarily.

Hospitals are administered by executive officers who are guided in their work by committees responsible for major decisions in respect of policy. The former may be medically qualified or lay. The latter are invariably mixed in the sense that they are composed of medical and lay members, the former representing the medical staff, the latter local interests. This committee directs the running of the hospital in the sense that it provides the wherewithals which enable the doctors to do their work. They are also responsible for providing the nursing and other services ancillary to medicine.

Every year each hospital reviews its expenditure, which is always rising, budgets in respect of running costs for the ensuing year, and makes recommendations as to its requirements in respect of new staff appointments, new equipment, and new buildings. These budgets are sent to the Regional Boards, England and Wales having been divided under the National Health Act into fifteen and Scotland into five regions from the point of view of hospital administration. The teaching hospital groups in England are directly responsible to the Minister.

The regional boards are responsible for the hospital services of their regions. They exercise no control over general practitioners, and local government is responsible for the public health services, the midwives, district nurses, health visitors, infant welfare services, vaccination, sanitation, etc. Again these boards consist of medical and lay members, and are run by medical or lay executive officers. The medical members of the Board represent the hospital interests and the lay members the life of the region. Every year these boards collate the budgets received from the hospitals and send their over-all recommendations to the Minister. Again and again they have to adjudicate on, and in point of fact sometimes to decide to reject the pet scheme put up by one hospital in favour of a different or even a similar scheme put up by another. Three hospitals, for example, say they would like to start a neuro-surgical unit or an accident department. But there is only the money, possibly only the need, for one. So the board now decides which hospital shall be allowed to start it, and get the money for it. This may be an extremely invidious decision.

Each year the Minister gets the budgets from all the regions and teaching hospital groups both in respect of maintaining services already existing and in respect of new developments. Each year, too, he learns from the government the proportion of the national income which they are prepared to devote to the Health Service, and therefore the hard facts relating to the amount of money which he will get to spend, both in respect of maintaining the Health Service at its present level and in respect of new developments. The Minister of course can never concede all the requests of all the regions. Rather, according to the degree of financial stringency prevailing, these have to be pared down, and again, just as the regional boards often have to refuse the request of one hospital and grant the request of another, so the Minister now lets one region go ahead with its cherished scheme but disallows the equally cherished plan of another. The country cannot afford both. He may allow a new unit for cardiac surgery, for instance, in region X, but not at present—of course he does not say never—in region Y. Further, the Minister's difficulties are often exacerbated by the fact that, as already pointed out, teaching hospitals and teaching hospital groups in England are directly responsible to him. So he may be in the embarrassing position of having to arbitrate between a teaching hospital group and a region in respect of some particular problem. Indeed, there may be a serious conflict between the interests of the university relating to teaching and research, and the requirements of the region in respect of the treatment of patients.

Whence it follows that the expenditure of money on health is not decided at the top by a Minister, advised by an expert lay and professional staff, in relation to how it could best be spent in order to maintain the health of the nation, as an innocent might suppose. The machinery of democracy does not work like that. Rather, whether money is spent on public health or health education (which has nothing to do with regional boards), for instance, or on homes for handicapped children or the aged (in which the teaching hospitals and universities are little interested), or on renal dialysis units and advanced surgery units (in which the teaching and the universities are very interested), or on general hospitals for the ordinary run of acute sick (in which the regional boards are mainly interested), depends on dog-fights in committees dominated by persuasive and outstanding personalities, local influence, politics and popular opinion prevailing at the time. Further, at the ministerial level, decisions are often of necessity to some extent political, and determined by the party in power. It is only necessary to think in terms of prescription charges to remember that. Is it better to charge for prescriptions, and spend more on hospitals, or abolish them and foot the drug bill at the cost of economizing in some other aspect of the Service? Decisions of this kind are really taken by Parliament and public opinion, rather than by the Minister.*

For money is short for the Health Service, and likely to get shorter as medicine advances and the cost of everything rises, particularly if everyone is to have modern medicine free on the State, and everyone is to be kept alive as far as possible regardless of the cost. So the question arises as to whether the expenses of the Health Service could be reduced without interfering with its efficiency. The re-introduction of prescription charges is a move in this direction. 'Hotel' charges for in-patients, particularly long-stay ones, would be another. A patient in hospital saves his expense of living at home. Those who can afford to pay should pay, many would maintain. Or, why not raise money on a sweepstake, as in the Irish Free State? The Church would oppose this. But the risk is that, unless something is done to save or raise money, the State may be forced into totalitarian methods.

It would be much cheaper to have district doctors to whom patients were forced to go, as in the medical services of the armed forces; cheaper to have hospitals which patients were compelled to enter rather than leaving them free to choose. It would be much cheaper to list drugs which may be prescribed, to forbid

---

* The Health Service, it must be remembered, was not started *de novo*. Rather, it took over three organizations already existing; the voluntary hospitals, the municipal hospitals, and general practice under the Insurance Act of 1912.

operations of doubtful value, to give guidance as to how far doctors should really strive to keep the aged and handicapped alive.

Any movement in this direction would be contrary to the spirit of British democracy, and remains correspondingly unlikely. Indeed, the strong point about the Health Service is the wide degree of freedom permitted within a service administered from Whitehall. A patient is free to choose his doctor. A doctor in general practice is under no obligation to undertake the treatment of a patient. Further, he is free to treat his patients as he thinks right, and as his conscience dictates. A Health Service patient can go into a Health Service hospital anywhere. All hospitals are free to plan ahead according to their own ideas within the limits of the control exercised by the Minister.

The future of the Health Service is hard to forecast. One thing alone seems certain. The cost of it is bound to continue to rise. So, as any move in the direction of totalitarian control is improbable, modification of it seems likely to come in three main directions. In the first place, a means test, and charges for luxury operations may well be forced upon it. In the second, more and more people may opt out of it by an extension of the insurance principle. Members of the salaried class are already tending to insure themselves so that they are treated as private patients when ill without being landed in great expense. Thirdly, some degree of reversion to the old voluntary hospital system is not altogether improbable. Some medical treatments are so expensive that the State cannot be expected to provide them, and few can afford to pay for them. For medicine of this kind, new voluntary hospitals, based on charity and dedicated to research, might rise phoenix-like out of the ashes of the old.

Teaching and research

Doctors have to be trained. This means that the right students must be selected. Then they must be taught. Further, medicine must progress. This means that their education should be against a background of research.

Selection is not easy. Many facets of personality are required, and the perfect doctor no more exists than the perfect horse. Intellectual ability up to a point is a clear prerequisite. But it is not the sole requirement. Other facets of character are also needed. A doctor must have moral integrity and the right sense of values. He must possess the ability to understand people and sympathize with them in their troubles, seeing their illnesses from their point of view, able to imagine what is going on in their bodies and in their minds. He must be prepared to carry responsibility, and possess the courage to take decisions. He must be careful and capable of sustained hard work, and also possess some sense of dedication, that is to say, willingness to sacrifice his life to it, at least to some extent. This is essential, particularly in general practice. On the other hand, he must be interested in his work as a branch of applied science. If he is interested in it only because it helps people, he will fail to keep up to date. If he is interested in it only as a branch of science, he will fail in judgment in human situations. General practice particularly demands this dual interest. Medicine ranges wide, however, and there is a niche somewhere for most types of mind, and for all to whom it appeals in any way and are possessed of honesty of purpose.

Practical medicine can only be learnt in the wards and out-patient department of a hospital. This means teaching on patients, and until 1948 this was carried out entirely in the medical schools of the voluntary hospitals. Patients were being treated free, and being used for teaching seemed a fair price for them to pay. That at least was the philosophy of it, and in point of fact reasonable restraint was exercised. Cases were selected with some regard for a patient's feelings, and teaching sessions were handled with tact. Few ever objected. When the National Health Service took over the hospitals, although the medical schools, now part of the university system of the country, carried on as before, the logic of this ceased to hold. Patients are now no longer being treated free. Rather, they are receiving something to which they are entitled as contributors to the Health Service, on the one hand, and as tax payers in a Welfare State on the other. But the Health Service cannot be maintained unless doctors are trained. It can therefore be argued instead that, as every patient is a beneficiary under the Health Service, it is his duty as a member of a Welfare State, on the principle of the happiness of the greatest number, to allow himself to be used for teaching in order to train doctors to look after other people.

The problem of progress by research is more difficult. Much medical research is, of course, carried out in the laboratory, and has either no connection with patients, or is only remotely connected with them. It is quite impersonal. Workers in the laboratory need to know nothing about the patient, and the patient himself knows nothing about what goes on in the laboratory. Further, many fundamental discoveries which have a wide application today, or will have one day, have been made, and are being made, by scientists with little knowledge of medicine and who have often been working in fields remote from it. (This applies to many recent recipients of Nobel prizes.) Much medical research, too, is merely observational, the recognition of diseases by their natural history. No ethical problems arise in this connection. Medical research only raises ethical problems when it concerns new methods of treatment which have to be tried out on patients.

Drugs are tested on animals first. The law now compels it, and there is unlikely to be any repetition of anything like the thalidomide disaster. But it is impossible to transpose the effects of drugs on animals to man with any great degree of certainty. Further, the risk of idiosyncrasy can never be ruled out. So, when new drugs are eventually tried out on patients, there is still some risk, and the long-term consequences of taking a drug can never be altogether foreseen even when no immediate unwanted side-effects ensue. The same considerations apply to progress in surgery. Operations are always tried out on animals whenever possible, and new techniques in surgery are always worked out on animals in the first instance. There are, of course, those who object to this. But that is probably a good thing. Opposition compels thought, and everyone would avoid pain and suffering to animals as far as possible. There are only two alternatives, however, to the use of animals; deliberate experiments on people, or letting people die. Most feel that man is 'of more value than many sparrows'.

A patient can volunteer to be experimented upon in the interests of either himself or of humanity. Recent transplant surgery has come very near to that, and many surgeons find new and difficult operations satisfying. They enjoy the technique of it, and surgery has a glamour that medicine largely lacks. It is performed in a theatre. It is necessary to dress up for it. There are spectators, and in the higher flights of it, the top surgeon leads an admiring team. Some surgeons are by nature exhibitionists, and even possess the 'I must be the first' mentality which can engender unfortunate inter-hospital and even international rivalry. Further, just as Gladstone, according to Disraeli, became 'inebriated by his own verbosity', so some surgeons, it seems, become inebriated by their own technical success, sometimes coming to view their achievements as likely to prove of greater value in relation to the needs of society as a whole than they really are. It is this infectious enthusiasm that, through modern channels of communication, and their frequent distortion of fact, has in the case of transplant surgery led a large section of the public to see it out of all proportion to its likely overall value in the practice of medicine in the future.

Surgery of this kind has attracted much publicity, but new drugs, modification of old operations, and new ones of a more ordinary kind, are always being tried out, as they must be if medicine is to progress, without either the public or the patient knowing anything about it. The public know nothing because neither the drug nor the operation is sufficiently sensational to be of news value. The patient knows nothing because the doctor is satisfied that there is a reasonable chance of the new drug or the new operation serving the patient better than any other drug or operation would serve him. If he does not feel that, in duty bound he asks his patient's consent to be experimented upon, for that is what his treatment now amounts to, pointing out, as he usually can, that this new drug or operation is likely to do him more good than any other remedy or course of action at his disposal at the moment. Further, it can be argued that as the patient of today benefits as the result of research on patients in the past, it is up to him to submit to clinical research, provided that there is a reasonable chance of him benefiting by it. In this way clinical medicine feels its way forwards. If the new drug or operation proves no improvement on its predecessors, a doctor does not try it again. If it is a success, he is encouraged to move further forwards in this new direction.

All medical research costs money, and this is derived from three main sources. Some is provided by the State out of the national income, and directed into the right channels by the Medical Research Council. Some is derived from legacies, individual gifts and contributions to charitable institutions, for example, the British Empire Cancer Campaign Fund. Research into pharmacology and the discovery of new drugs is mainly financed by the manufacturing chemists. For the link between chemical composition and pharmacological action is seldom yet apparent, and research in this field is still mainly empirical, the chemical firms spending large sums of money on producing a succession of substances which *might* prove useful in medical practice, work of a kind which university departments cannot afford to undertake. Only occasionally do the former strike lucky, and then get the money spent on much unproductive work back by putting this new drug on the market at a price well above its actual cost of production. This precipitates an odd situation. Modern drugs are of necessity often expensive, and raise the cost of the Health Service. But research of this financially risky kind could hardly be taken over by the State, these firms nationalized like the railways and the mines.

When a doctor, as opposed to a firm, discovers a substance of therapeutic value, he is not allowed, according to the ethical code of his profession, to exploit or make money out of it. So when Banting and Best discovered insulin, the Therapeutic Substances Act was carried, and by international co-operation comparable legislation introduced in other countries. Insulin can only be manufactured by firms licensed to do so under this Act. By this means the standard and the price of insulin have been controlled, and no one, not even the discoverers, or makers, made money out of it, except, of course, the reasonable profit allowed to firms licensed to manufacture it. Since then a number of other substances useful in medicine have been added to a list, of substances, the manufacture of which is controlled by the Act, notably vitamin B_{12}, used in the treatment of hyperchromic, or as it was once called, pernicious anaemia.

* * *

The decision as to what to do about a patient may be difficult for technical reasons. The diagnosis cannot be established for certain, or it is impossible to forecast the treatment which will work the best. It may also be difficult for human reasons. Is it really worthwhile doing this or that, or indeed doing anything, in view of the patient's age, the kind of life which the only form of treatment might permit, the suffering it will prolong, or the strain it will impose on his relatives? Decisions of this kind depend on human judgment. There are no scientific answers. They demand a sense of values of which science can take no account, and that is why clinical medicine can never become, in spite of what so many seem to think, a science. In theory the general practitioner, who treats his patients in their own environment, is clearly the man to take these decisions. But he may have lost touch with his patient when he was taken into hospital, and in these days he has become a specialist himself, a specialist in general practice, and in consequence is often no better qualified to evaluate the medical worthwhileness of doing what the specialists advise, than the specialists are in a position to evaluate the worthwhileness of doing what they advise in relation to the patient's home circumstances. But *his* patient is now in *their* hands, and usually consents to whatever they advise with the result that there is some risk sometimes that what is done is determined more by what *can* be done technically rather than by what *should* be done in the light of human considerations.*

* Unfortunately the gulf between the work of the general practitioner and that of the specialist is widening as hospital medicine becomes increasingly technical and correspondingly mechanized.

CHAPTER X

PROBLEMS RELATING TO DEATH

Enabling to live—Keeping alive—Modern dilemma—The moral problem—Letting die—The legal position—Management of the dying.

Everyone born into this world, although in the rush of the business of life it is largely forgotten, or anyhow kept well out of mind, is born into it to die. 'Think not the doom of man reversed for thee.' So, besides getting people well, part of a doctor's work is to shepherd people out of life.

Enabling to live

Man often cheats nature, and prevents life starting. He sometimes terminates pregnancy six months before an infant would be born. On the other side of the balance-sheet he can frequently enable a child to live which otherwise would not have long survived its birth. This statement applies particularly to infants born prematurely; and to those with malformation of the heart or defects of the nervous system.

Until recently any infant born before the end of the eighth month of pregnancy, and weighing less than 2 lb., rarely lived, and again and again this statement held true of quadruplets and quintuplets, sometimes due to taking fertility pills, which attract so much morbid publicity. For children of multiple pregnancies tend to be born prematurely and under-weight. But in these days it is often possible to keep infants born weighing less than 2 lb. alive. Evidence is, however, accumulating to suggest that, although the lesser degrees of prematurity do not seem to matter, extreme degrees of it result in the mind failing to develop as well as it might have done had the child not been born so soon.

These children grow up of lower intelligence than brothers and sisters not born until full term. The brain, it would appear, is not ready for an extra-uterine existence until about the eighth month of pregnancy. The environment of the incubator does not always equate with that maintained *in utero*.

When twins are born conjoined, although cases are on record that have lived like that for years, the risk of separating them is usually taken. When their union is by skin, or by skin and muscle, separation is easy. Both continue living. When they are conjoined in respect of some vital organ, the nervous system, the circulation or the gastro-intestinal tract, the life of one is now risked or sacrificed in order to maintain that of the other.

Many congenital malformations of the heart can be satis-factorily repaired. These fall into two groups. In one the infant looks normal at birth because a sufficient supply of oxygenated blood reaches its tissues. The diagnosis is made later, and the malformation is repaired when the need arises. In the other the infant turns blue at once because the circulation of blood through its lungs is insufficient due to narrowing of the pul-monary valve and a patent interventricular septum. An infant of this kind is severely handicapped, but the defect can often be repaired at the appropriate age after its exact nature has been ascertained. Many blue babies grow up into adult life.

The repair of malformations of the nervous system is less satis-factory. In about one in a thousand cases the spinal canal fails to close (spina bifida) leading to protusion (meningocele) of the meninges, due to the pressure of the fluid within, through the unclosed gap at that point. This must be repaired within a few hours or at least a day or two of birth. This saves life, but does not remedy the defect of development of the spinal cord with which it is often associated. Sometimes there is no defect. Then, to all intents and purposes, after the operation the infant is back to what it ought to be. More often the lower part of the cord has failed to develop properly and, in spite of a successful operation, as judged from outward appearances, the child, as it grows up, proves to be paralysed in its legs. Moreover, as the innervation of the bladder depends on reflexes through the lower part of the cord, many of these children suffer from incontinence, and sometimes die of urinary infection. Spina bifida and meningocele are also frequently associated with failure of the normal development of the ventricular system of the brain, and this, again in consequence of the pressure of the spinal fluid, leads to hydrocephalus. This condition, which also occurs unassociated with spina bifida, necessitates a repair operation. But it is by no means always successful, and children, hydrocephalic on this account, often fail to develop normally in mind or, at any rate, remain of low I.Q.

A cretin, if diagnosed in time and fed with thyroid, as has already been seen, grows up into a near-normal child. Infants born with pyloric stenosis can be saved by incising the pyloric valve which regulates the passage of food out of the stomach. But these constitute an outstanding exception to a general rule. Most children with congenital disorders of function can be helped little either by medicine or by surgery. Nothing radical can be done, for example, about cystic disease of the pancreas or kidneys, haemophilia, inborn errors of metabolism, the myopathies, mental deficiency, mongolism, and many other congential conditions. Until recently most of them, like so many normal children, died of broncho-pneumonia.

Keeping alive

In these days, however, as the result of the introduction of antibiotics during the last war, most seriously handicapped children can now be kept alive, not necessarily to live out a normal span of human existence—many are too handicapped for that—but to live much longer than they would have otherwise. Some of them, particularly the children of the well-to-do, are kept tucked away at home, sometimes much-loved pets, at others a source of embarrassment to parents and distasteful to their brothers and sisters. Others, including most with the more serious defects, are cared for in special homes manned by dedicated staff. The mentally retarded are taught in special schools.

At the other end of life the picture has changed too, and changed for much the same reasons: namely, the use of antibiotics in the treatment of pneumonia. An elderly man or woman who, for any reason, needs to be put to bed, no longer dies of hypostatic pneumonia, as it was called then, almost as a matter of course. Rather, old people now live on, sometimes only to develop senile dementia, the health of the body sometimes far outlasting that of the mind.

The same holds true in respect of the middle years of life in the sense that a large number of middle-aged people are now kept alive much longer than they would otherwise live. Again this is largely due to antibiotics, the main single factor in the therapeutic revolution which has transformed the face of medical practice. The bedridden suffering from rheumatic and ischaemic heart disease, the effects of strokes due to high blood pressure or arterial degeneration, paralysis agitans, chronic bronchitis and emphysema, the chronic rheumatic diseases, and many other conditions, live much longer than they did a few decades ago. Further, blood transfusion and closed circuit methods of anaesthesia now permit extensive operations on bones and joints, on heart and lungs, on spinal cord and brain. The chronic sick, to use the official nomenclature of administrative medicine, now occupy an increasing proportion of the hospital beds in the country.

Further, although the risk of serious accidents has mounted, the extent to which the severely injured can be kept alive has steadily increased, partly due to antibiotics, safe blood transfusion and better anaesthesia, and partly due to skilled nursing care, particularly in the case of injuries to the brain and spinal cord. These are mainly due to car and motor cycle accidents.

A fractured spine with complete division of the cord in its mid-dorsal region leads to paralysis of both legs (paraplegia) and anaesthesia to all forms of sensation below that level for life. For nerve fibres, once divided, never regenerate *within* the nervous system. But these patients soon learn to hoist themselves into and get about in wheelchairs, and they have full use of their hands with which to help themselves. Others are more unfortunate still. High spinal injuries, the commonest cause of which is diving accidents, lead to tetraplegia. The patient is now paralysed in all four limbs, although he can usually move his shoulders and, depending on the exact level of the lesion, use his triceps to extend his elbows to help himself a bit. Many ingenious devices are available to enable him to help himself still further, and a man in this state has even learned to drive a special motor car. Most of these are cared for in special centres, as the patient can only go home if a near relative, prepared to dedicate her life to his service, is available. Looking after a tetraplegic is a full-time occupation. The married are sometimes able to satisfy the other partner, and a tetraplegic has actually given birth to a child.

The extent to which men with severe head injuries recover after long periods of unconsciousness during which, until not long ago, they would certainly have died of bronchopneumonia, is remarkable. Many of them return to work or, anyhow, go back to work of some kind eventually. But the longer a man with a severe head injury lies unconscious, the less likely is he to recover consciousness, and if and when he does recover it, the less likely is he ever to be his normal self again.

Modern dilemma

The attitude of man to death varies according to race, culture and religion.

In the East, individual life is held of no great importance. The attitude to death is essentially fatalistic. It is of little significance. In certain circumstances suicide is even a duty, as with the Japanese in the last world war. In the communist countries, too, the State rather than the individual is held of primary importance, and a man must be prepared to sacrifice his life for it.

According to Christian teaching individual life matters, each one just as much as every other. Premature death is an evil; suicide cowardly; sudden death a disaster. They allow no time or opportunity to repent. 'From battle, murder and sudden death, good Lord deliver us.' So runs the Litany of the Church of England. The concept of hell and eternal punishment, responsible at one time for so much fear of death, is outmoded, but by failure to live as he should, a man can lose his soul. He renounces his inborn claim to immortality. The religious man must therefore necessarily remain to some extent afraid of death. Will it be the turning point of life? Or is he, as the result of the way he has lived, condemned to oblivion? It was for this reason that Dr. Johnson, in spite of all his wisdom, was so afraid of it. He feared to meet his Maker.

The non-believer is beset by no such fears. Some live in vague hope, feeling that at death the truth will be revealed; and that all will then be well somehow, somewhere, in a way that man cannot comprehend. Others are more afraid of dying than of death. Further, it now so much easier for anyone to shut death and all that out of the mind than it was, say, sixty years ago. Parents no longer expect to lose some of their children, as did Victorian and Edwardian mothers, and in these days, when relatives do die, they often leave this world in hospital or in a geriatric institution, and so, largely out of sight, sometimes even out of mind, rather than at home. In consequence most people manage to keep death and dying well out of their lives, much as they manage to keep the killing and death of the animals, which they eat daily, well out of their minds. In consequence they live largely unprepared for it.

Faced with death men want to live. The survival instinct is strong, and human beings have always looked to doctors to protect them and their's from it. 'Doctor, can't something be done?' is the cry of relatives in distress, and the long-established tradition of medical practice is for a doctor to strive to keep his patient alive, and enable even the unwanted child to live. So, although recent advances in medical science now enable him to restore many people to normal or anyhow reasonable health and to relieve pain and suffering as never before, he sometimes finds himself in the uncomfortable position of keeping a handicapped child alive to remain a burden on its family or the State, or a man or woman alive merely to suffer for no apparent benefit to himself or herself, or to anybody else. He may find himself keeping an old person alive who, it seems to him, on all ordinary standards has lived long enough already, and in whose case commonsense would seem to say that it would be much better to withhold any further treatment, and let him or her depart this life in peace.

Society incorporated into the State is in a similar and, in a kind of way, even worse predicament. Keeping premature infants alive, and operations for congenital defects, cost money. Homes for spastic, epileptic, mongol and other handicapped children, and special schools for them, cost money. Institutions for the aged and the incurable, centres for spinal and head injuries, artificial kidney units, resuscitation teams in hospitals, all cost money. This is a hard fact, and two problems arise. Firstly, to what extent should money be spent in the interests of *one* patient when the same large sum, as in the transplantation of an organ, could have been used to help many others in some other way? Secondly, is the proportion of the national income which the government allocates to the maintenance of health being spent to the best advantage of society? Might not some of it be better spent, at least so it can be argued, not on homes for hopelessly handicapped children, not on artificial kidney units, not even on geriatric institutions for the aged, but in striving to promote the health and happiness of Bentham's greatest number? It could be spent on intensified research into this or that, on more efficient hospitals, on expansion of the social services, on health education. It could be spent in fields outside medicine altogether, for instance, on higher pensions for old people or on making safer roads and thereby reducing the incidence of head and spinal injuries. It might be used to aid the backward countries, to help in famine areas, to save the lives of refugees. In short, are modern medicine and the resources of the State being used and directed at the present time in the best interests of humanity?

These are hard questions, and of the kind to which it is always tempting to turn a blind eye, and carry on as humanity and sentiment dictate regardless of the ultimate consequences. It is always the path of least resistance to shirk them. Further, they raise questions of principle and faith on which there is no general agreement, the answer which one man gives to them, and the attitude which he adopts towards them in practice, often cutting right across the conscience and practice of, and causing grave offence to, the convictions of another.

The moral problem

According to Christian teaching life is a gift, and the doctor is under a moral obligation to keep his patient alive as long as he can by means put into his hands. Suicide, too, is sin. A man has been given his life, and it is not for him to opt out of it. But even Roman Catholic moralists hold that a doctor is only under an obligation to keep his patient alive as long as life can be *reasonably* maintained. Further, he need only use ordinary methods. These are those easily available. The extraordinary include those still in the experimental stage, of great expense, or not yet generally accepted.

According to the scientific interpretation of man the body is the product of blind chance, and the mind developed on it ceases to exist with its death. Life, on this view, is not a gift but an accident, and when the question of keeping alive arises the doctor should take into account the utilitarian principle of the health and happiness of the greatest number. On this view, too, suicide is not necessarily an offence. Rather, by taking his own life, or refusing treatment which would prolong it uselessly, a man can relieve his family or the State of a heavy burden.

These are extreme views. The former puts the individual first. The latter exalts the over-riding interest of the State. Between them all shades of opinion exist, but the practice of medicine inclines traditionally to the first. A doctor's primary allegiance is to his patient, and totalitarianism in the organization of medical practice is to be resisted. But there is no escape from the fact that, as the result of the rapidly increasing power of medicine, a doctor is now often compelled to make up his mind whether a certain course of action which will only prolong life miserably is seriously worthwhile, not only in terms of the kind of life it will permit his patient, but also in relation to the strain it will inevitably impose on relatives and the cost to them or to society incorporated into the State. No longer can the doctor always treat his patient in isolation. He is a member of society, and has a moral duty in relation to it. Further, under the Health Service the doctor is not only the servant of his patient. He is in part in a sense a servant of the State.

In theory the patient should decide whether he really wants to be kept alive a little longer, or perhaps kept alive in some unhappy state much longer, a burden on his family or society. In theory he should face up to the ethics of the situation himself. In practice this is seldom practicable. He is too ill, or not sufficiently intelligent, and even if he is in possession of his faculties and sufficiently intelligent, his decision is determined by the way in which the pro's and con's for action or inaction are put to him by his doctor. A decision, although sometimes seemingly a patient's, is in fact usually his doctor's. Nor can near relatives be asked to take decisions of this kind for much the same reason. Either they do not know enough about medicine, or cannot visualize the situations which will soon arise, or they are too emotionally involved. When this is tried, again and again the same reply comes back: 'Doctor, you know best.' And in point of fact he invariably does. Doctors alone can, and therefore must, take these decisions.⟩

Most would agree, however, that in deciding the question of letting his patient die quietly versus striving to keep him alive a little longer, a doctor should handle him according to what he, his patient, believes or does not believe, quite apart from what he, his doctor, believes or does not believe himself. If his patient is a Roman Catholic, for instance, he must try to keep him alive even when his own commonsense as a free thinker dictates that it would really be more sensible to let him depart. Roman Catholic doctors, however, and some Anglicans, feel under a moral obligation to handle their free-thinking patients according to their own principles. This is both unsatisfactory and insufficiently realized.

The responsibility of doctors in these matters is now very great, as in these days, to an increasing extent, they are compelled to decide what ought to be done in situations of this kind. There is no one else who can take these decisions, and right decisions clearly depend on getting the right men and women into the profession; humanizing the early stages of medical education; the maintenance of a high standard of general practice; and on close co-operation between general practitioners, who treat their patients in their own environment, and hospital consulting staff who treat them mainly out of it. Again and again between them they must arbitrate, to the best of their judgment and ability, between the tradition of their profession to keep alive, on the one hand, and the suffering of their patients and the interests of society as reflected in the family or the wider one of society, on the other. When in doubt, however, they must always err on the side of striving to keep alive. The public relationships of the medical profession are of paramount importance. Loss of confidence of the public in it would be a social disaster. A doctor's training should enable him to judge when to let nature take its course. But the tradition that he is a trustee of life must at all costs be maintained.

Letting die

In point of fact no doctor always 'strives', to quote the oft-quoted words of Clough, 'officiously to keep alive'. There is a natural limit to what he feels he should do, although often not to what he might do, and at a certain point there comes a moment at which he throws in his hand. Further, if a man is dying of some untreatable condition, diagnosed up to accepted standards of certainty, he does not make any attempt to keep him alive just a little longer except in special circumstances; the impending return of a near relative from abroad or the necessity for him to take some great decision. It is usually immaterial whether he dies on Tuesday or Friday, this week or next. But there are border-line cases, and the decision between letting die and striving to keep alive may have to be taken deliberately.

The handicapped child within the family circle, sometimes a family pet, at other times a family burden, presents a difficult problem. When pneumonia would remove it from the human scene, how hard should the doctor really strive to keep it alive? Some do so, regardless of the human cost. Others are guided by its degree of wantedness, its own potential future, the happiness of all concerned, and the feelings and religion of its parents, remembering that a mother may want to keep it for her own sake, rather than for its, the same problem as faces a vet when someone wants to keep a pet alive for purely sentimental reasons.

A man may be so severely injured in an accident that the chances of any semblance of useful life being left to him are so remote that it seems best to commonsense that he should die. (In wartime, decisions of this kind are taken again and again.) In a less severe case the doctor strives to keep him alive, assuming that his patient will be able to adapt himself to the disability with which he will be left. This may be very great. He may be left blind, emasculated, paralysed in both legs or quadriplegic. But many such live on more or less happily for years. They are glad, they say, to have been kept alive.

Severe head injuries leading to unconsciousness present a difficult problem. Again a doctor assumes that his patient wants to live, but must doubt that he would wish to continue to live a

wreck of his former mental self. So, if there is evidence of extensive cerebral damage, or a man has been unconscious for a long
time and his electro-encephalogram has ceased to record waves
for a sufficient time, then ventilation of the lungs, if respiration
is being artificially maintained, is sometimes switched off, or his
water intake gradually whithheld so that his body, now that his
mind has gone, dies of the accumulation of the end products of its
own metabolism. But these cases are of necessity looked after by
a team of nurses and doctors, and many consciences may have
to be squared before this can be done.

A man in full possession of his senses, when told that he has
cancer, may deliberately refuse the treatment which might save,
and would anyhow probably prolong, his life. Whether this is
suicide is a question of definition. Whether it is moral turns on
the circumstances of his life and the nature of his case, and it is
not for his doctor to pass judgment on that. Far more often a
man in this position clutches at any straw, and whenever there is
a chance of radical cure or prolongation of useful life by a combination of excision, endocrine and X-ray therapy, this is always
advised. Palliative surgery, such as colostomy in inoperable
carcinoma of the colon, and oophorectomy, adrenalectomy and
even hypophysectomy in carcinoma of the breast, is a different
matter. Procedures of this kind seldom prolong life more than a
few months, or a year or so at the most. They are in fact extraordinary methods of treatment which most doctors agree should
not be employed except for special reasons. No one need be
expected to endure too much merely to live just a little longer.

The sudden collapse of a middle-aged or elderly man due to a
coronary attack with cessation of heart beat and respiration
demands an immediate decision. The doctor on the spot—he will
not accomplish much unless he or a trained layman happens to
be there—makes up his mind at once as to whether to attempt
resuscitation. In a relatively young man it is always attempted.
The circulation is maintained by cardiac massage, and respiration by the mouth to mouth method, while he is rushed to hospital where his heart can sometimes be re-started. In many old
men, on the other hand, it is clearly not worthwhile. Cardiac
infarction is a good 'way out', and any attempt is unlikely to
succeed. Old people are not being resuscitated repeatedly in

general practice by the 'kiss of life' and cardiac massage as is sometimes supposed. And, if the doctor does succeed, it is often questionably worth it. His patient has been recalled to life only to die a few weeks or months later of the same condition. Therefore, while in these circumstances a doctor may make a show of doing something—public opinion expects it or he may think in terms of what the coroner might say in court—he may act without any real intent to succeed. Age is relative, however, and there are border-line cases. That is the difficulty. But many an elderly man in these days really feels, that, if he should have a severe coronary attack, with the result that he is on a good bus for the next world, he would not wish to be forcibly pulled off it. Some talk of carrying their wishes in this eventuality—and perhaps in the event of being admitted to hospital on account of a severe head injury—on their person. But it is questionable whether these would be legally binding on the doctors.

The legal position

The legal position of a doctor who deliberately withholds treatment which would, or anyhow might, prolong life, is even less clear than his moral position. For statute law lags behind technical advances in medical practice, and common law is now faced with many unprecedented situations.

Once a doctor embarks on the treatment of a patient, whether he has been chosen personally by him, or treats him in the capacity of a doctor selected by a hospital to treat its patients, he is under an obligation to show such ability as can reasonably be expected of an average doctor, or if he is a specialist, of an average specialist. He is under a similar obligation, if he undertakes the treatment of a patient voluntarily, taking charge, for instance, of a person found unconscious or of a man who has just had a coronary attack. He is under no legal obligation to do it. In this country he is not even under an obligation to pull a drowning child out of the water. But public opinion would look askance at him, and the coroner would make defamatory remarks about him in court, if he did not do what is generally regarded as his social duty. If now, having taken on a professional obligation of this kind, he fails in it in some way, he can be found guilty of negligence, and becomes liable for damages. If his patient dies as the result of it, and his negligence was gross, he can be found guilty of manslaughter. So the question arises as to whether letting his patient die, rather than helping him to live, can sometimes be interpreted as doing his best for him; and, if it cannot, whether a doctor who withholds surgery in a gross congenital abnormality or antibiotics in the case of a mongol child or elderly person dying of pneumonia, or deliberately switches off the machine ventilating the lungs in a case of severe head injury, when the mind is 'dead' but the body still alive, is guilty of manslaughter or even of murder.

The answer to this question is uncertain until a case of this kind has been brought to court to create common law, or the medical profession make representations to the government who introduce and carry legislation creating statute law, in regard to the matter. But the average doctor makes a distinction in his own mind between letting nature take its course by withholding treatment, for instance, not giving antibiotics or a blood transfusion, and deliberately calling off treatment, for instance, keeping an unconscious patient alive by mechanical ventilation of his lungs and then stopping it deliberately. The latter seems to him too like killing. So he naturally hesitates to start lines of treatment which, for this reason, he finds difficult to stop. Whether this distinction on his part will prove to have validity in law will also only be decided when a case is brought to court.

Management of the dying

When a man is dying, the question may arise as to whether he should be told, but it does not do so anything like so often as might have been expected. It does not arise, for instance, in the case of a man destined to die suddenly. His doctor may know, of course, and often does know, that this may happen. In high blood pressure, for example, it is possible to give a statistical prognosis. But the individual is a law unto himself. While one man with a pressure of a certain figure dies soon, another of the same age with the same pressure lives on for many years, and he is likely to be scared enough, in need of reassurance rather than of being frightened into being overcareful. Nor does the problem arise in acute infection. A man is usually too ill to be told, or the doctor himself does not know whether his patient will recover until he is past telling. Nor does it often arise in the commonest cause of death—progressive failure of cardio-respiratory function. The patient knows that his heart is failing, and the doctor does not know when the end will come much better than the patient does himself. A man, too, who has had a stroke or a coronary attack lives in the knowledge that he may get another. There is no point in reminding him of that. In fact the question of telling versus not telling only seriously arises when a man, who thinks he is in health, or until recently felt in it, is discovered to be suffering from some lethal condition such as inoperable cancer.

Some people in these circumstances are told as soon as the diagnosis has been established. Their position in society, their family responsibilities, or their religion demands it. Many men of character, although they do not subscribe to any orthodox belief, can take it, and are better told. In other people, particularly in those where faith does not exist to hold the fort, a doctor may be less certain as to what to do, and it is for this reason that doctors in general are often accused of not telling their patients often enough, or of not telling them soon enough, in short of not being sufficiently candid with them, particularly in and by a generation which expects to know and be told about everything. There is something in this accusation. But many a man who maintains that he expects to be told when he is dying, when that time comes, never asks questions, and clearly prefers, consciously or unconsciously, to slip out of the world unknowingly. Indeed, many manage to repress the realization of their impending death, even the most intelligent men succeeding sometimes, their approaching end being obvious to everyone except to they themselves. So a man is sometimes best left to live clear of the shadow; better kept in false hope rather than getting to know too soon. The nearest and most responsible relative is, of course, told. His advice is often needed, and his co-operation essential, if a conspiracy of silence is to be maintained. The risk is being found out, and the patient losing all confidence in his doctor. But in practice this seldom happens. And doctors on the whole find it better not to tell many patients too soon, often not in fact until a point is reached in their downward progress when it becomes a relief to them to know that they are dying.

In most cases the body fails before the mind, but pain and mental distress can usually both be relieved by means of drugs, notably morphine and heroin, which detach the mind from reality, and the modern tranquillizers, which reduce emotional reactions. Common humanity dictates that, in these circumstances, these should be given and continued in sufficient quantity, although this often means stepping up the dose as the patient develops tolerance. Drugs given on this scale cloud the mind, and heroin particularly leads to alteration of personality. So the Catholic and Anglican Churches insist that the patient must be told that he is dying before they are started, and his mind lapses into fantasy. Drugs of this kind, given in this way and for this purpose, do not, however, as is commonly and erroneously supposed, shorten life. Rather, the relief of pain effected by them slows down bodily activity, and the patient tends to live longer with the result that they may much increase the physical and emotional strain on relatives and friends. Further, it is difficult both to give dangerous drugs on this scale, or nurse these patients, in their own homes, and a man dying in this way often blocks a hospital bed for a very long time indeed.

In other cases the mind fails before the body. A person loses his speech, so that he cannot communicate with his friends, or, as the result of widespread arteriosclerotic changes in his brain, mind and personality depart, leaving the body living on alone. The latter do not suffer. But their relatives suffer much, and these patients sometimes live on for years a burden to their families or the State.

Under criminal law, as it stands today, euthanasia, which literally means 'good dying', that is to say, dying well—a personal challenge—but a word which has come to mean the deliberate shortening of life in order to prevent further pain or suffering, or to relieve society of a burden, is, of course, illegal and, if perpetrated, would be murder. But a somewhat anomalous situation has been created by the Act of 1961 which abolished suicide from the category of a felony. A man is in fact now at liberty in law to take his own life, and faced with permanent paralysis or death from cancer can commit, if that is the right word, voluntary euthanasia. This is still generally regarded as cowardly as the result of generations of conditioning of opinion in this direction by Christian teaching. But it seems a strange verdict. If a man is expected to rise superior to his other instincts, he should be admired for rising superior to his instinct to live at all costs, particularly living on as a burden on his relatives, society, and the State. Captain Oates, who deliberately walked out into the blizzard, goes down to history as 'a very gallant gentleman'.

Under the same Act, a doctor is specifically debarred from deliberately putting the means to that end into his patient's hands. If a doctor knew that a patient of his in hospital intended to take his own life, he would be legally responsible for stopping him doing it, his overall care being temporarily in his hands. In private practice, providing his patient was in his right mind, his liability would end at discussing it with him. Modification of the law in order to legalize euthanasia, as above defined, has in fact often been, and is now again being suggested. The Roman Catholic and Anglican Churches continue to stand adamant against it, and for the same reason as when faced with so many other medical issues. Death belongs to God, and it is not for man to take His decisions into human hands. The other Churches also see purpose in life, and in general hold it to be a man's duty to try to stick it out to the end, rather than opt out of it at will. Secular opinion, on the other hand, although it realizes that any law legalizing euthanasia would be difficult to draft in such a way as to prevent abuse and avoid imposing an intolerable burden of painful decision on society, cannot see why, in certain circumstances at any rate, man should consistently continue to deny to man that mercy that he so readily concedes to an animal.

*　　*　　*

The power of medicine over human lives and minds has increased, is increasing and is bound to increase still further. That is certain. At the same time it is fast becoming clear that, if this new-found power is to continue to be used to relieve suffering, and the money available for the promotion of health is to be spent in the best interests of society, doctors must exercise restraint and protect their patients sometimes from some of the things which science now enables them to do. A thing must not be done *just because* it *can* be done. Technical achievement must not become our God. The concept of personal integrity in relation to society must also become the corner-stone of all health education. This seems particularly important. Every man holds his health in his own hands to some extent. He is also responsible in varying degrees, directly and indirectly, for that of other people.

Finally, we all must learn to adopt a more aggressive, anyhow a more *resigned*, attitude to the natural phenomenon of death than that which generally prevails at present. We must not strive too hard against it, and in so doing force the doctor's hand. 'Addiction to life', wrote C. S. Lewis, 'is no more respectable than addiction to drugs.' Death, the great experiment, is not the greatest of all evils, even if there is no meaning in human existence:

> *He there does now enjoy eternal rest*
> *And happy ease, which thou doest want and crave,*
> *And further from it daily wanderest:*
> *What if some little payne the passage have,*
> *That makes frayle flesh to feare the bitter wave,*
> *Is not short payne well borne, that brings long ease,*
> *And layes the soule to sleepe in quiet grave*
> *Sleepe after toyle, port after stormie seas,*
> *Ease after warre, death after life, does greatly please.**

* Spenser, *The Faerie Queene*, Canto IX, 40.

INDEX

Abortion, 141
Achondroplasia, 109
A.C.T.H., 35
Addison's disease, 166
Adrenal glands, 35, 128, 166
Agnosticism, 78
Air, pollution of, 114
Alcohol, 116, 133, 135
Allergy, 119
Amino-acids, 30 32
Amphetamine, 136
Anaemia, aplastic, 113, 121; iron deficiency, 111; haemolytic, 166; hyperchromic, 188; due to haemorrhage, 112
Anaesthetics, 115
Analgesics, 134
Anatomy Act, 174
Angina, 125
Anglican opinion, 140, 198, 204, 205
Animal experiments, 186
Anorexia nervosa, 100
Antibiotics, 165, 192; resistance to, 165
Antibodies, 117, 119
Antilymphocyctic serum, 171
Antitoxin, 117, 165
Aphasia, 55, 126
Appendicitis, 165
Arnold, Matthew, 13, 91
Arsenic, 115
Arteriosclerosis, 125
Artificial insemination, 147; kidney, 169
Assessment of fitness, 129
Asthma, 119, 128

Atomic explosion, 114, 123
Auto-allergic disease, 120
Autonomic, 37, 94, 98

Barbiturates, 115, 165
Barium, radioactive, 114
Bed-wetting, 100
Behaviour, 61, 99; animal, 19
Benign growth, 122
Bentham, Jeremy, 87, 153
Beri-beri, 111
Birth, 34
Blood groups, 26; pressure, 42, 122; transfusion, 170
Blue babies, 191
Body and mind, 61, 80
Body, embryology of, 29; physiology of, 17; segmental origin of, 41; self-adapting, 18; self-maintaining, 17; self-protecting, 18; self-regulating, 17; self-repairing, 18
Body-mind, 15, 59, 64; relationship, 85, 127, 128
Bone, growth of, 34, 72, 92; grafts, 169
Brain, parts of, 37; transplantation of, 173
Breast, carcinoma of, 167, 200
Breathing, 42
Broca's area, 55
Bronchitis, 132
Broncho-pneumonia, 192
Burns, 113

Calorie requirement, 111

Cancer, 122; fear of, 94; treatment of, 167, 200
Cannabis, 116, 135
Carbon monoxide, 114
Carcinogens, 123
Carcinoma, 122; treatment of, 167, 200
Cardiac infarction, 128, 168; massage, 167
Cardio-inhibitory centre, 42
Castration, surgical, 167; physiological, 167
Cataract, 126, 167
Causation, 31
Cell division, 23, 34
Centre, cardio-inhibitory, 42; vasomotor, 42; vomiting, 42
Centres, emotional, 52, 64
Cerebellum, 45, 67
Cerebral haemorrhage, 126; syphilis, 103, 176; thrombosis, 126
Cervix, carcinoma of, 157
Chance, 24, 31, 79
Chemotherapeutic agents, 165
Chicken-pox, 118
Childhood, 69
Childlessness, 147
Chlorine, 114
Choice, conscious, 61, 87; physiological, 44
Christianity, 77, 87, 139, 140, 194, 196
Chromosomes, 23; abnormalities of, 109
Chronic sick, 193
Churches, World Council of, 140
Cirrhosis, 116, 134
Claustrophobia, 99
Cleft palate, 166
Climacteric, 126
Clinical trials, 186; diagnosis, 159
Clough, 199
Cocaine, 136
Colour blindness, 109
Commandments, 87
Common cold, 118; law, 131; sense, 80

Compulsion neurosis, 99
Compulsory restraint, 149
Computer, 43, 62, 67
Conditioning, 60
Conflict, 95
Congenital defects, 108, 121; treatment of, 166, 191
Conscience, 71, 77
Consciousness, 20, 50, 61; dawn of, 64; mystery of, 61, 84; stage of, 62
Constitutional weakness, 92
Contraceptives, 139
Conversion hysteria, 100
Co-ordination, 43, 45
Corneal grafting, 170, 174
Coronary disease, 125, 132, 171; obstruction, 168; thrombosis, 125, 200, 203
Corpus callosum, 49; luteum, 36
Cortex, auditory, 48; motor, 45; sensory, 47; silent, 55; visual, 47
Cortical activity, 51
Cortisone, 115, 129
Cretinism, 35, 166
Criminal responsibility, 152
Curare, 115, 165
Cystic disease, of kidneys, 192; of pancreas, 192

Dangerous Drugs Act, 137
Dead body, law relating to, 174
Deaf mutism, 67,
Deafness, 126
Death, attitude to, 194, 206; definition of, 174; fear of, 195; mechanism of, 173; surivival after, 80
Defaecation, 42
Deficiency disease, 111
Degeneration, 125
Dehydration, 111, 164
Delirium tremens, 134
Dementia, senile, 126
Depression, 93; endogenous, 104; pyschogenic, 103; somatogenic, 103
de Quincey, 137

Descartes, René, 15
Describing v. explaining, 22, 58, 83
Determinism, 79
Development, 34; embryonic, 29; muscular, 73; pyscho-sexual, 72, 146; psycho-somatic, 63
Diabetes, 121, 166
Diagnosis, clinical, 159; laboratory, 161; mistakes in, 162
Dickens, Charles, 106, 109
Digitalis, 115
Diphtheria, 117, 165
Disease, causes of, 108; concept of, 130; functional and organic, 108
Disseminated sclerosis, 20
Dissociation, electrolytic, 38; mental, 97, 100, 105
Divorce, 147
D.N.A., 20, 28
Doctor-patient relationship, 156, 197
Donors, supply of, 175
Double helix, 21
Dreams, 52, 63, 99, 179
Drug addiction, 101, 114, 136
Dualism, 85
Duodenal ulcer, 121
Dying, management of, 202

Eating, 132
Education, 70; religious, 71; sex, 71
Egalitarianism, 92
Electric convulsion therapy, 176
Electro-encephalogram, 51, 52, 200
Embryology of body, 29; of personality, 65
Emotion, 61, 93, 157
Emotional centres, 52, 64, 127; states, 103
Emphysema, 126
Empiricism, 86
Enabling to live, 190
End organs, 41
Endocrine glands, 34, 41
Endocrines, see Hormones
Energy, 15; mental, 96
Entropy, 19

Epilepsy, 102
Eunuchism, 113
Euthanasia, 204
Evangelicism, 77, 153
Evolution, 31, 79
Evolutionary sequence, 91
Excitement, see Mania
Existentialism, 86
Explaining v. describing, 22, 58, 83
Extroversion, 94

Factory Act, 153
Faith, 89; healing, 157
Familial disease, 26
Fantasy, 67, 70
Fear, 94, 162
Feed back principle, 37
Fertilization, 24, 139, 149
Fibrillation, 168
Fidelity, 140
Final common path, 45
Firms, pharmaceutical, 188
Fitness, assessment of, 129
F.L.H., 36, 71
Foot and mouth disease, 118
Free will, 80, 86, 151; and the law, 81
Freeze drying, 170
Freud, Sigmund, 53, 178
Frigidity, 98
Frontal cortex, 55, 67
F.S.H., 36, 71
Functional instability, 93
Functional and organic disease, 108

Gage, Phineas, 55
Gametes, see Germ cells
Gangrene, 125
Gastric ulcer, 121, 167
General practitioner, 156, 180, 185, 189, 198
Genes, 23, 124
Genetic defects, 108; plan for body, 27; for mind, 60
George III, 109
Germ cells, 23; formation of, 24
German measles, 143

Glands, 34, 41
Goitre, 121
Gonadotropic hormones, 36, 71
Grafting, 169, 174

Haemodialysis, 169
Haemolytic anaemia, 166
Haemophilia, 109
Hallucinations, 106, 116, 136
Happiness, 62, 88
Hare lip, 166
Hay fever, 119
Head injuries, 194, 199
Health, definition of, 92; education,
   138, 154, 206; Service, 155, 180–4
Hearing, 47
Heart, congenital malformation of,
   171, 191; transplantation of, 171;
   beat, cessation of, 167; block,
   168; disease, 125, 132, 171; failure,
   120, 123
Heat stroke, 113
Height, 72, 92
Heroin, 116, 135, 204
Herpes zoster, 118
High blood pressure, 124
Homicide Act, 152
Homoeopathy, 158
Homosexuality, 73, 146, 179
Hormones, 34
Hospital, admission to, 163; doc-
   tors, 158, 180, 189, 198
Hospitals, administration of, 181;
   municipal, 155; voluntary, 155,
   185
Human relationships, 130
Human Tissue Act, 174
Huntingdon's chorea, 107
Hydrocephalus, 192
Hydrocyanic acid, 115
Hypertension, malignant, 125
Hypnotics, 134
Hypnotism, 84, 164, 178
Hypothalamus, 52
Hysteria, 99

Identification, 68

Idiosyncrasy, 116
Immunity, 119
Immuno-suppressive drugs, 166, 171
Impotence, 98
Infancy, 66
Infarction, 168
Infection, 116; acute, 117, 202;
   chronic, 118; reaction to, 117;
   staphylococcal, 117; streptococcal,
   117; syphilitic, 118; treatment of,
   165; virus, 118
Inflammation, 165
Influenza, 118
Injury, 112, 164, 199
Instinct, 59, 61
Insulin, 35, 121, 188; shock therapy,
   176
Integrity, 88, 138, 140, 144, 206
Intellect, 53
Intersex, 110
Introversion, 94
Intuition, 86
Investigations, 162
Ionizing radiation, 113, 144
Isoniazid, 165

Jaundice, 115, 160
Johnson, Dr. Samuel, 78, 81, 194
Joints, artificial, 167

Kant, Immanuel, 91
Keeping alive, 192
Kidney disease, see Nephritis; failure,
   see Renal; transplantation, 170
Knowledge, 86
Knox, Ronald, 82

Laboratory diagnosis, 162
Laryngitis, 160
Larynx, transplantation of, 172
Law, common, 131; natural, 87;
   statute, 131
Lead poisoning, 115
Letting die, 199
Leucotomy, 57, 176
Leukaemia, 113, 122
Lewis, C. S., 206

Liberty, 134, 135, 136, 149
Lichen planus, 121
Life, chemical basis of, 20; criteria
of, 20; futility of, 96; origin of, 32
Liver, transplantation of, 172
Love, 62
L.S.D., 116, 136
Lunacy, 149; and Mental Treat-
ment Act, 150
Lung, carcinoma of, 114, 124, 132;
transplantation of, 172

Macbeth, Lady, 99
Machine, the human, 15–20, 22
Malignant growth, 122; treatment
of, 167
Malignant hypertension, 125
Malnutrition, 111, 164
Man, management of dying, 202;
nature of, 77; origin of, 31; posi-
tion of, 79
Mania, 104
Manipulation, 159
Marajuana, 135
Marriage, 145; guidance, 155
Marx, Karl, 77
Masturbation, 71
Materialism, 78, 85
Mathematics, 83
Measles, 118; German, 116
Medical Research Council, 188
Medicine, mechanisation of, 189
Memory, 53, 63, 69
Mendel's Law, 26
Meningocele, 191
Menopause, 113, 126
Menstruation, 36
Mental disease, prevention of, 177
Mental energy, 62; Health Acts,
150; states, diagnosis of, 107, 161;
stress, 128
Metabolism, errors of, 109, 192
Metaphysics, 85
Methyl alcohol, 115
Micturition, 42
Mind, explanation of, 57; genetics
of, 59; nature of, 84; universal, 84

Minister of Health, 144, 182
Miracles, 158
Mistakes in diagnosis, 162
Modern dilemma, 194
Molecular accidents, 30, 129; bio-
logy, 21, 28
Mongolism, 109
Moral philosophy, 87; values, 71
Morphine, 116, 135, 204
Motor cortex, 61
Movement, co-ordination of, 43, 45;
reflex, 41; voluntary, 45
Multiple pregnancies, 190
Mumps, 118
Municipal hospitals, 155
Muscle, varieties of, 40; contraction
of, 16
Mutation, 30, 123, 129
Myopathy, cardiac, 171
Mysticism, 86
Myxoedema, 66, 121
Myxomatosis, 118

National Insurance Act, 155; For-
mulary, 180
Natural selection, 31
Nature, laws of, 79
Nephritis, 120, 168
Nerve cells, 37; fibres, 37; impulses,
38
Nervous system, 37; formation of,
30; shock, 128
Nervousness, 94
Neuritis, peripheral, 116
Neurones, 40
Neurosis, 97; obsessional, 96; com-
pulsion, 99
Neurotic reactions, 98
New growth, 122; cause of, 123;
treatment of, 167, 200
Night blindness, 111
Nucleoprotein, 20, 29
Nucleotides, 32

Oates, Capt., 205
Obesity, 92, 132
Objectivism, 86

Obsession, 96
Oestrogen, 37, 72
Opium, 116, 135
Organ transplantation, ethics of, 173; legality of, 174
Organic disease, 129
Organs, preservation of, 175
Osteo-arthritis, 126
Osteopathy, 158
Otosclerosis, 126
Ova, 23
Ovarian cycle, *see* Sexual cycle
Oxygen requirement, 111

Pacemaker, artificial, 168
Pain, 160, 164; psychogenic, 94; relief of, 204
Palliative surgery, 200
Paraplegia, 191, 193
Parapsychology, 84
Parathyroid, 35
Pathological processes, 161
Pathways, sensory, 47; motor, 45
Patients, sorting of, 181
Paupers, 155
Penicillin, 165
Perception, 46
Peripheral neuritis, 134
Personal integrity, 88, 138, 140, 144, 206
Personality, 63
Perversion, 102
Pharmacy and Poisons Act, 134
Philosophy, 84; moral, 87
Phosgene, 114
Physical injury, 112, 164
Pituitary, 29, 34, 37, 71, 127; hormones, 34
Plan, genetic, 27, 60
Planets, 32
Plants, 16
Plastic surgery, 167, 170
Pleasure, 61, 66
Pneumonia, 192; virus, 118
Poisoning, 114, 134; treatment of, 165
Poisons List, 136

Poliomyelitis, 118
Polycythaemia, 121
Poor Law, 155
Porphyria, 109
Position, sense of, 45
Pragmatism, 88
Pregnancy, multiple, 190; prevention of, 139, 190; termination of, 141, 144, 190
Prematurity, 190
Prescribing, 180
Preventive medicine, 153
Progesterone, 36, 139
Promiscuity, 138, 140
Prostate, carcinoma of, 167
Protein as antigen, 119; requirement, 111
Psittacosis, 118
Psoriasis, 121
Psychedelic drugs, 106, 116, 136
Psychiatric treatment, 175
Psychoanalysis, 53, 63, 178; existential, 86
Psychopathic behaviour, 88, 101, 110
Psychoses, 103; functional, 104-5; organic, 176; treatment of, 176
Psychosexual development, 72, 146
Psychosomatic concept, 64; development, 65; disease, 126
Psychotherapy, 17
Puberty, 36, 71, 73, 102
Public health, 153
Purpose, 81, 91

Radium, 167
Rationalism, 86
Real world, 50, 82
Reception order, 150
Reflex action, 41
Regional Boards, 181
Rejection, 169
Religion, 76, 91
Renal failure, 120
Repression, 97, 99
Research, 186
Resistance to antibiotics, 165

Respiration, artificial, 167
Respiratory centre, 42
Responsibility, criminal, 151
Restraint, compulsory, 205
Reticulo-activating system, 44, 50, 61
Rheumatism, 120
Rheumatoid arthritis, 120
Rickets, 111, 164
R.N.A., 28
Rogue cells, 123
Roman Catholicism, 96, 139, 141, 158, 196, 198, 204, 205
Routine examination, 157

Sarcoma, 122
Sartre, Jean-Paul, 86
Schizophrenia, 106, 176
School, 70; medical service, 154
Science, 79, 197
Scurvy, 111
Semi-circular canals, 45
Sensation, 47
Sensory cortex, 61
Sex, determination of, 27; chromosomes, 26; hormones, 71, 167; instinct, 72
Sexual characteristics, 37, 144; cycle, 36
Sexuality, 37, 71, 138
Shakespeare, William, 88, 126
Skin grafting, 169
Sleep, 51, 63
Small pox, 118
Smell, 44
Smoking, 132
Social psychiatry, 177; services, 154
Somatopsychic disease, 127
Soul, 81, 141
Speech centre, 67
Spenser, Edmund, 206
Spermatogenesis, 36
Spermatozoa, 23
Spherocytosis, 109
Spina bifida, 191
Spinal cord, 37; nerves, 37
Spine, fracture of, 193

Spiritual vision, 77, 90
State, 153, 155; intervention of, 153; medicine, 183, 188
Statute law, 131
Sterilization, 144
Steroids, 171
Stone formation, 121
S.T.P., 116, 136
Streptococcus, 120, 165
Strokes, 126, 203
Strychnine, 165
Students, selection of, 185
Subconscious, 63
Subjectivism, 86
Sublimation, 96
Suicide, 197, 204
Sulphonamides, 165
Sulphur dioxide, 114
Suprarenal, see Adrenal glands
Surface-volume law, 66, 111
Surgeons, 187
Surgery, legality of, 145; palliative, 201; progress in, 187; transplant, 169, 186
Surgical excision, 167
Synaptic junctions, 40
Syphilis, 118; cerebral, 103, 176; congenital, 116

Talking, 67
Teaching, 185, 198; Hospital Groups, 181
Teenage problems, 74
Telepathy, 84
Temporal lobe, 54
Termination of pregnancy, 141, 145
Test-tube babies, 149
Testosterone, 37, 172
Tetanus, 117, 165
Tetraplegia, 193
Thalamus, 49, 61, 66
Thalidomide, 186
Theology, 78
Therapeutic Substances Act, 188
Therapeutics, 164
Thermodynamics, 19
Thyrotoxicosis, 166

Thyrotropic hormone, 37
Thyroxine, 34, 37
Time, sense of, 49, 61; schedule, 28, 34
Tissue banks, 170
Tonsilitis, 120
Toxins, 117
Tranquillizers, 115, 134, 204
Transcendental, 78, 89
Transplant surgery, 169
Tuberculosis, 120, 165
Twins, conjoined, 191; identical, 30

Ulcerative colitis, 121, 167
Uncertainty principle, 80
Unconsciousness, 194, 199
Urinary incontinence, 191
Utilitarianism, 77, 87

Values, 83, 89; moral, 71
Variation, 30

Vaso-motor centre, 42
Venereal disease, 140
Virus hepatitis, 137, 169; pneumonia, 118
Viruses, 118, 123
Vision, 47; failing, 126; spiritual, 77, 90
Visual cortex, 47
Vital force, 20, 28
Vitalism, 20, 28
Vitamin B, 117, 134, 176; B$_{12}$, 188
Voluntary hospitals, 155, 184, 185
Vomiting, 42; centre, 42

Walking, 67
Welfare State, 185
Wells, H. G., 106
Will, 54, 63, 66
Wish fulfilment, 100

X-ray sickness, 113
X-rays, 123, 167